A HEALER'S JOURNEY TO INTUITIVE KNOWING

"This work invites an awakening to the depth of our shared humanity; entices us to pay attention to subtle, as well as non-subtle, phenomena; and engages in some of Krieger's favorite phenomena, such as synchronicity, serendipity, and even miracles. Even though nursing is the origin of Therapeutic Touch and Krieger's beginning work, this text is not only for nurses. This work moves to embrace, invite, and include all healers in numerous disciplines—any and all energy lightworkers involved in concepts and practices of holism, wholeness, energy medicine, energy healing, nonphysical distant healing, and so on. This writing is guided by the energy of love and a conscious intentionality to serve as an agent of healing—of wholeness. A great addition to any healer's library."

JEAN WATSON, PH.D., R.N., FOUNDER AND DIRECTOR OF
THE WATSON CARING SCIENCE INSTITUTE

"In this final offering from Dolores Krieger, her journey from discovery to deepening to actual wisdom is generously shared. *A Healer's Journey to Intuitive Knowing* is the distillation of more than five decades of exploration, practice, and teaching of Therapeutic Touch. Beyond method and technique, she traces the flow of healing back to its source—compassion and the ever responsive Inner Self—and speaks to the essence of healing and self-knowledge. Over time the great teachers like Dolores seem to grow in their simplicity. In this book she offers a guidance that begins with consciousness and ends with that same consciousness magnified by an intuitive knowing born from the compassionate commitment to heal. This is a necessary book for anyone drawn to healing and the deepening self-awareness it demands."

Tim Boyd, international president of
the Theosophical Society Adyar

"Dolores Krieger provides us with insights into the intricacies of energetic healing, which the general public often finds difficult to comprehend. In great detail and in layman's terms she manages to dissect the anatomy of a healer and of energetic healing in a way I have not come across before in my 25-year career."

Tjitze de Jong, author of
Energetic Cellular Healing and Cancer

"It is amazing and encouraging that the founders of Therapeutic Touch (TT) successfully carved a path to work alongside mainstream medicine and managed to spread their network throughout America and beyond. Their many healing stories—addressing physical, mental, and emotional issues—support my own clinical research findings that professional standards of training ensure safe and highly effective holistic healing that can be delivered in less than half an hour. Dolores's book is a wonderful testament to the dedication of TT healers, whose fine work improves people's lives—and, along the way, their own, too."

Sandy Edwards, author of
Spiritual Healing in Hospitals and Clinics

"The emphasis on resonance, frequencies, and the practitioner's ability to go into a state of stability and regulation relates powerfully to some of the newer body-based healing modalities, such as Somatic Experiencing. The body-mind state of the practitioner is paramount in these practices, as it is here in this wonderful book. Dolores's Therapeutic Touch approach draws on elements of physical and subtle realities that empower the healing process that arises within the relationship of two people—the healer and the healed."

Nancy J. Napier, LMFT, author of
Sacred Practices for Conscious Living

A HEALER'S JOURNEY TO INTUITIVE KNOWING

THE HEART OF THERAPEUTIC TOUCH

DOLORES KRIEGER, Ph.D., R.N.
Edited by Julia Graham Benkofsky-Webb

Bear & Company
Rochester, Vermont

Bear & Company
One Park Street
Rochester, Vermont 05767
www.BearandCompanyBooks.com

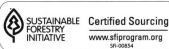

Text stock is SFI certified

Bear & Company is a division of Inner Traditions International

Cataloging-in-Publication Data for this title is available from the Library of Congress

ISBN 978-1-59143-393-4 (print)
ISBN 978-1-59143-394-1 (ebook)

Printed and bound in the United States by Lake Book Manufacturing, Inc. The text stock is SFI certified. The Sustainable Forestry Initiative® program promotes sustainable forest management.

10 9 8 7 6 5 4 3 2 1

Text design and layout by Priscilla Baker
This book was typeset in Garamond Premier Pro with Optima, Futura, and Gill Sans used as display typefaces
Illustrations on pages 19, 32, and 235 courtesy of Charles Elkind, charliescards11@yahoo.com

To send correspondence to the editor of this book, mail a first-class letter to the editor c/o Inner Traditions • Bear & Company, One Park Street, Rochester, VT 05767, and we will forward the communication, or contact Julia Graham Benkofsky-Webb directly at kalaoa@hawaii.rr.com or PO Box 1657, Kailua-Kona, HI 96745.

*With deepest gratitude on the part of
the global Therapeutic Touch community
to our teachers
Dora van Gelder Kunz
&
Dolores Krieger
(Dolores was fond of using the term D^2
in reference to the two of them)*

When you center yourself in meditation you consciously experience wholeness—your undivided unity with everything that exists. You see yourself, as well as the people with whom you have relationships, as part of that immense wholeness. It is in this sense that we interact with one another most authentically. On the personal level we are always separated from one another by the barriers of the ego, but these barriers do not exist at that deeper level. When we are able to detach ourselves from personal interest, we can reach out to people in a much more enduring way.

DORA VAN GELDER KUNZ, *THE PERSONAL AURA*

The prime characteristics of energy are that it flows or is continuous as it moves through space, that its flow has a coherence or rhythm, and that is has the capacity to do work. Its flow has been described on a continuum from slow to fast, strong to weak, unimpeded to congested, tenuous to thick, or quiet to tumultuous, depending upon the situation. Its rhythm has been characterized as steady or irregular, in harmony or unharmonious, in sync or disorganized.

DOLORES KRIEGER, *THERAPEUTIC TOUCH AS TRANSPERSONAL HEALING*

We don't have energy fields.
We are energy fields.

MARTHA ROGERS, R.N., PH.D.,
NURSE HEALERS PROFESSIONAL
ASSOCIATES CONFERENCE, TORONTO, 1990

Contents

PART I

THE WAY OF THE HEALER
Exploring the Consciousness of Therapeutic Touch

PART 2

EXPERIENTIAL KNOWLEDGE OF HEALING
Therapeutic Touch Exploratory Studies

❧

A Healer's Journey
Path of Transformation

By David Spangler

It was my mother who introduced me to Dolores Krieger and the work of Therapeutic Touch (TT). Mom was a registered nurse, dedicated to healing and always open to finding new ways to serve the patients under her care. Over the years of her career she became less and less satisfied with a purely Western allopathic approach to medicine and began to explore other healing modalities. Generally this was to expand her own knowledge, as she usually worked in hospitals and doctors' offices that were not open to anything outside current medical orthodoxies. But occasionally opportunities arose in which she could try "something different" to help a patient.

It was in this context that she discovered Therapeutic Touch. Unfortunately, by the time that she did, she had retired, but I remember how excited she was by it. Here, she felt, was a simple, practical method that any nurse could use in quiet, unobtrusive ways to help patients in an otherwise allopathic medical setting that was not open to alternative approaches. She was even more excited when she learned that TT was being taught in nursing schools. Discovering this made her feel proud to be part of a profession that was expanding its frontiers to enhance its own ability to serve.

When I went home to visit, Mom shared her excitement about TT with me, which of course raised my own interest in this approach. This was at a time in my life when I was traveling a great deal, speaking at conferences and holding workshops in various parts of the country, which brought me into contact with many people exploring new ways of living more holistic lives and creating more wholeness in the society around them. Having had my awareness of Therapeutic Touch heightened by my mother, I was alert to paying attention when someone I met mentioned TT or was actually practicing it.

It was in this context that I had the pleasure of meeting the author of this book, Dolores Krieger, while speaking at a convention. On another occasion I had the equal pleasure of meeting her partner in developing TT, Dora Kunz, who was, at the time I met her, president of the Theosophical Society in America. Both instances were brief, unfortunately, and I would have treasured an opportunity to have spent more time with either of them. I particularly felt a kindred spirit in Dolores, which is why it is an honor to write this foreword to her book.

I like to say that we live in two ecologies. Both are all around us, but one is tangible and visible—the physical world we see and with which we interact every day. The other is just as real but is less tangible, less visible, and often in our materialistic society viewed as nonexistent, a figment of our imaginations. This is a nonphysical—or what I call "subtle"—ecosystem, filled with forces, energies, and lives that are as much a vital component of our living planet as the physical world around us. Knowledge of this invisible, subtle dimension has been categorized in various ways: religious, mystical, shamanic, psychological, even magical. I think of it simply as "the other half of Earth's ecology," an integral part of our planet's wholeness.

As a species, we actually have a great deal of knowledge and insight about this subtle dimension, gained over millennia of human experience and exploration. In our time and culture, much, if not most, of this is scattered, lost, or kept in a fragmented state as different insights remain the proprietary and separated knowledge of one group or another.

Recovering, restoring, renovating, and releasing humanity's collective wisdom about the subtle realms is one of the great projects of our time.

However, an even more important project, I believe, is that of exploring and understanding how the two great ecosystems of our world—the physical and the nonphysical—interact with and affect each other. I would even go so far as to say that our fate as humanity and even the fate of our world as we know it depend on this understanding, for it is nothing less than understanding the wholeness of our planet, how we fit into this wholeness, and how we must act to support and enhance it.

It is not only a deeper and more comprehensive understanding of the interplay of life and energy between the subtle and physical worlds that we need. We also need the tools, the holistic applications, the practices that are born of this interaction and draw their efficacy from it. To approach the world only from a physical standpoint or only from a spiritual, mystical, transcendent, subtle aspect is not sufficient; we need both. We need the alchemical blending and wholeness of both.

This is where Dolores's work with Therapeutic Touch is so important, as it is just such a holistic tool. It honors who we are as inhabitants of the world in its wholeness, and not just as physical beings. It proudly and effectively works right on this boundary where the two ecosystems meet and interact. This is not surprising, as we ourselves are an embodiment of that meeting ground and that interaction. Part of us is obviously physical, but part of us is not. Whether we call it the psyche, Inner Self, soul, mind, or something else, we all experience a subjective, intangible aspect that cannot be limited to or fully defined by our physical form. And what better way to demonstrate this wholeness than through a healing art?

This book, like Dolores's life and work, presents in clear terms this meeting place of the two planetary ecosystems. It offers a holistic paradigm of what it means to be a human being participating in a living planet. This by itself would make this book worthwhile.

But Dolores has gone much further here than simply presenting an abstract, theoretical picture of the interaction of physical and nonphysical realities. What is so wonderful about this book is that it takes us into the experience of the healer who is using TT, giving us a step-by-step look at each stage of the process. Like Dolores herself it is down-to-earth and practical, seeking to put Therapeutic Touch onto a solid theoretical foundation but also showing how it is lived.

Laboratory experiments have tried to show the reality of various forms of subtle-energy healing, such as TT, but have often failed to provide substantive evidence that convinces the mind of an orthodox skeptic. This is because a process like TT doesn't live in a laboratory. It is an organic, lived process that takes a great many variables into account, from the energy field and psychological (and physiological) state of the patient to the energetic nature of the surrounding environment, and more. All of this is dynamically synthesized and distilled by the healer who is in the midst of it all, not doing something *to* someone else but participating *with* the patient and with the whole of life of which we are all a part.

This is what is so difficult, if not impossible, to replicate in the sterile environment of a laboratory in which an experiment tries to exclude all the variables except the one under study. Life excludes nothing; it is filled with variables that interact with each other, and it's in this arena that TT operates and must be understood.

It is this participatory, living, holistic element that Dolores communicates so well in this book, giving readers almost a hands-on experience of what is happening. We are invited into the skin of the healer, allowing Therapeutic Touch to become part of our lives as well. In so doing we are learning not just a healing art, but the art of being itself.

Not all of us are called to be healers, but I believe we are all called to be agents of wholeness in our world. Dolores embodied this. In this book she gives us a gift of insight and empowerment that enables us to be the same.

Issaquah, Washington
2020

David Spangler is an internationally renowned spiritual explorer, codirector of the Findhorn Foundation from 1970–1973, and author of more than thirty books, including *Working with Subtle Energies*.

Adventures in Healing with Dee

It was a gentle Montana morning before sunrise at the end of May 2019, and I was on my way from Columbia Falls to the Kalispell airport. In my previous three days in Montana I had made my last visit to my teacher, Dolores Krieger, who was then under twenty-four-hour care at her home. We knew she was in her final days, although she would briefly rally in early June, even hosting a merry gathering on her deck complete with fudgesicles. On the night before my flight I had sat with Dee, holding her hand as she fell asleep. It was a precious gift to be able to spend time with her at this stage of her life. As I flew home that morning I carried with me a daunting responsibility: Dee had designated me as the editor of her "one more book" that she had been working on for a couple of years. Her amazing stores of energy had been carrying her forward even though, as she said in her ninety-seventh year, "What used to take me a day, takes me a week," and she had resisted suggestions for changes from her loyal manuscript readers. But now, at the end, I had learned that she was asking for some assistance.

The purpose of Therapeutic Touch is to bring order to a disordered vital-energy field, therefore the healer must be calm when she responds to the call. Energy from the universal healing field is offered unconditionally to the person in need. As Dora Kunz often reminded us, "Your purpose is to bring order where there is disorder, not to end the suffering so much as to bring order." This teaching is ingrained within each of us who has chosen Therapeutic Touch as our healing path. There are a number of excellent books about the TT method written by my teacher and others, but the perspective of this new work was to be that of the person in the role of healer. It was envisioned to be accessible to practitioners of other disciplines of energy medicine—presented as an exploration of the reality experienced by the healer from within these therapeutic interactions.

Dee had been providing me with many adventures (in both the outer and inner worlds) since we first met at Camp Indralaya, Eastsound, Washington, in 1991. It was a privilege to attend the invitational workshops held there each June, to study with Dee and Dora and many experienced TT folks. In 1995 I served as coordinator of the conference of Nurse Healers Professional Associates (now Therapeutic Touch International) held in Kona, Hawaii, near my home. Dee had a long-standing connection with the Hawaiian Islands, so it was a treat to provide the means for her to travel to the volcano on our island, where, she said, she had some "unfinished business with Madame Pele," goddess of the volcano. I never learned what the business was but she must have completed it, as throughout the years she often expressed appreciation for having had the opportunity.

Dee loved the phenomena of synchronicity and serendipity. Both of these were in play when one of my daughters was in a school just a short distance from Dee's home in Columbia Falls. This provided me with the opportunity for some unanticipated visits with her. I was touched when Dee, a lifelong vegetarian, prepared a chicken for dinner with my carnivore daughter. Many could cite examples of similar kindnesses over the years.

During the first decade of the twenty-first century, until 2009, I spent a number of years assisting Dee in the planning and teaching of the TT workshops at Indralaya, which required us to be in weekly phone contact. This period also included years of working with her on the book *The Spiritual Dimension of Therapeutic Touch,* published by Bear & Company, which consisted of transcriptions of talks by Dora Kunz that had been recorded at Indralaya on Orcas Island, Washington, and at Pumpkin Hollow Farm in New York. This project involved several work sessions in both Hawaii and Montana. At times, Dee could demonstrate a remarkable ability to regard her life's work with irreverence and humor, and during the writing of that book she was so delighted when spell check converted "crown chakra" to "clown chakra" that she developed a skit based on that misinterpretation.

There had been so many memorable experiences. By June 2019 I was feeling the weight of the task Dee had assigned. On all the other adventures she had been my guide—encouraging, prodding, cautioning—as we shared ideas and planned events. However, I was not to be alone in carrying this weight. Help appeared immediately in the form of Sandy Matheny and Dr. Pat Cole, who have walked each step of this journey with me. Their support has been invaluable. Friends and TT colleagues of Dee, these two Montana gals had been a consistent presence with our teacher for more than a decade—a physical presence that those of us who were far-flung geographically could not offer. Our trio has remained united in our commitment to helping birth this exploration of healers' experiences to be shared with our TT family and beyond, with colleagues in related fields.

As will become evident through hearing all the voices in this book, TT people don't allow time and space to stand in our way when we need to connect with one another. Through the months of preparing the manuscript, sometimes I have felt Dee standing behind me or whispering in my ear.

Many of us know how untempered a comment could be from Dolores Krieger. Often upon seeing me after some time, she would declare, "You look exhausted!" That memory makes me smile now.

Thank you, Dee—for all the joys and sorrows, your ferocious mind, and your tender heart. And for teaching us all the ways we can bring order from disorder. Deepest bow of gratitude.

JULIA GRAHAM BENKOFSKY-WEBB
KONA, HAWAII
2020

Introduction

Over the course of history, healing has been one of humankind's higher functions, leaving its mark as a spiritual practice throughout more than 10,000 years of human civilization. All of the major religions include healing as one of their expressions of spirituality, and so it should not come as a surprise that there are innumerable ways to practice healing. Considering such a long list of healing practices, one wonders at the commonality among them. It is interesting that although the practice of healing is older than civilization, no one has ever clearly defined the experience of the healer engaged in the healing moment; it remains ineffable.

In Therapeutic Touch (TT) healing is perceived as a humanization of energy that conveys the sense of order and the power of compassion to body systems that are fatigued, in trauma, imbalanced, in a state of disrepair, or in final transition. The crux of this mode of healing is that Therapeutic Touch facilitates vital-energy (*pranic*) flow by bringing order to dysfunctional physical and psychodynamic systems of sentient beings. These actions are done within a transpersonal frame, and it may be that the experience of being in this realm of beyond-the-personal is what prompts many TT therapists to embrace this method of energy healing as a personal spiritual practice.

The entry point into the Therapeutic Touch process itself is a state of centered consciousness. Centering is taking a moment to connect within to a place of silence and stillness, setting aside one's own troubles and concerns to find an inner peace. This state is sustained throughout the entirety of the healing session, while the therapist simultaneously offers a variety of TT skills where appropriate. As one continues to practice Therapeutic Touch, it becomes evident that it is this sustained state of consciousness that nurtures and empowers the therapist.

This book is offered as an exploration of the process of healing, concentrating on one aspect—the perspective of the person in the role of healer. The experience under scrutiny is the flow of energy during the session between the therapist and the person seeking healing. In the exploration of this personal knowing, a compelling finding is the relationship of these interior experiences to one another in a strikingly intelligent, centrally integrated manner. In the context of healing, this constant shift of consciousness is the platform for Therapeutic Touch, which we are using as a model for healing in general. It is a heroic leap that lifts the person whose life is committed to helping or healing those in need from the more common acts of daily living to compassionate engagement in the healing process. The two spheres of action are worlds apart. What, one wonders, urges the healer to aspire to such a high calling?

It is difficult to know with certainty the source or impetus of such aspiration. A hint seems to be that the fountainhead for such high calling is sourced in a different realm from that limited by the space-time we normally inhabit. Across time and in many and diverse cultures, historical records have told and retold the story. It has been the way of the compassionate healer engaged in the helping or healing of others who has been able to safely mount that high path with admirable perseverance and surety.

In observing a Therapeutic Touch session it is initially difficult to realize that an experience that appears to be so direct and simple could call out significantly advanced and complex shifts in consciousness in the therapist. However, it rapidly becomes obvious to the involved therapist herself that it is not as simple as it looks; in fact, its complexity is as deep as the therapist's understanding will allow.

It is possible to view the healing process in terms of two general aspects: the theoretical content, research, and clinical studies of the process itself; and the experiential knowledge that comes from the inter-action between therapist and patient, which leads the therapist to a personal knowing. (These are explored in more depth in chapter 6.)

These two aspects are coupled with many other ongoing functions, the whole engagement growing synergistically to rapidly foster personal growth experiences. For instance, as the healer is feeling compassionate concern and helping the "healee,"* the inner work that is simultane-ously occurring in her heart chakra proceeds at more subtle levels. Also in this act of interiority, both the theoretical and experiential aspects of healing may become more clearly understood and integrated. In addi-tion, as the healer matures in the practice of TT, the entire complex of these aspects serves to unify, expedite, and enhance the subtle, evolving, interior processing that sets the stage for the enactment of the transper-sonal in her life.

At this writing, more than fifty years have passed since my col-league Dora Kunz and I began the development of Therapeutic Touch. Much of what our culture now takes for granted was as yet unknown at that time. The act of healing and its rationale relied heavily on a reli-gious frame of reference, and science could not find an adequate context for it. Therapeutic Touch challenged religious traditions of healing by asserting its most basic assumption: healing is a natural human potential that can be actualized under appropriate conditions. This assumption declares that the healer is not a specially chosen person who is divinely anointed. Therapeutic Touch also challenges the scientific perspective in that it "works" even though we still do not fully understand how subtle energies are transferred from healer to the one seeking healing.

In developing Therapeutic Touch Dora Kunz and I used every means of exploration at our disposal. Probably the first avenue of that initial development of TT arose out of our experiential knowledge as we began to realize that we could help people who were ill, and ana-lyzed what we had done so that we could continue to help others. Much of that early work stemmed from our many observations of other

---

*Throughout this book the person seeking healing—the healing partner—will frequently be referred to as the healee, and for ease of use, male pronouns will be applied. —*Editor*

acknowledged healers at work. Dora observed from her unusual, world-class clairvoyant perceptions; mine were from a more ordinary frame of reference that was now and again gifted with a fortunate insight. It was from this considered blending of those observations of expert healers and our own experiences that we began to develop our basic suppositions of what was transpiring under our hands during the healing sessions. This was not always a straightforward, logical process. Under the best circumstances it was flashes of tested intuitions and thoughtful sensitization to inner promptings that helped us leap forward, even in the face of a more generally accepted logic that might point in another direction. However, our saving grace has been that we have always been willing to test notions before presenting them. From the early days we always emphasized to our students: take nothing on faith but test the ideas in your own Laboratory of the Self.

It was out of this amalgam that we developed our theories about the healing process, most of which we have had the opportunity to retest over the years. The persistent, driving force of our uncomplicated desire to help those in need energized our grasp of the reality of the transpersonal infrastructure of the Therapeutic Touch process, and it is at the transpersonal level of the personality that the most potent work of the TT process may be glimpsed.

Additionally, from the beginning the development of Therapeutic Touch was sponsored by universities, hospitals, and health professions in the United States and later by TT therapists, community health agencies, and other institutions in a large number of the countries of the world. Having that academic and professional support in the background of Therapeutic Touch required that we develop the curriculum in a formal manner that spoke to the validity and reliability of the theoretical content. The theoretical content could then be tested and graded, and so over time it was established that Therapeutic Touch was not only teachable but also could be learned. With the development of standards of practice and evaluation tools, Therapeutic Touch quickly became a pioneer in the formal entrance and acceptance of optional therapies in the arena of higher education, as well as in adult education, life studies, and at-a-distance education.

How will healing evolve in the next decades and centuries of human history? It is indeed heartening to view the increase in numbers of medical doctors adopting complementary medicine disciplines. Since the early days when Dora and I were observing the acknowledged healers, much has changed in healthcare options. Only one example of many is the Andrew Weil Center for Integrative Medicine in Arizona.

The concept that the ability to facilitate healing for another person is literally in our hands has become widely accepted. The idea that we can use our consciousness to offer healing energetically at a remote distance from the recipient is no longer regarded as implausible.

I have always been fascinated with predictions and ruminations about the future. It is not difficult to see that our time is at the leading age of multiple worldwide changes that are focalizing, converging, and combining in previously unimagined ways, resulting in an era of unprecedented events. Future consciousness is considered to be the total set of percipient abilities, processes, and experiences humans use in dealing with the future. Indeed, it is future consciousness that has propelled human evolution throughout the ages.

Under the press of what has been called the New Enlightenment, we are beginning to realize that the problems looming in our future are so incredibly complex that they need the minds of several people to envision their new calculus. Fostering a mindset of inquiry, as we concomitantly exercise future consciousness, will open us to alternative answers to our problems. This focus will give access to the infinitude of possible expressions of our aspirations for meeting the future-conscious development of the Therapeutic Touch process as this era unfolds. We are in a unique time that permits untold possibilities for personal transformation. Consequently, if we are ready for it, the universe will be behind our efforts toward radical change in each individual's life path and in our resolute quest for deeper insights into helping or healing those in need.

I foresee that with the increasing presence of virtual reality and artificial intelligence—our far-reaching world of hi-tech—there will continue to be a place for the high-touch of Therapeutic Touch and related energetic therapies. Healing, the most humane of all human attributes, is a worthy counterbalance—perhaps even companion—to many of the technologies of the New Enlightenment. The compassionate practice of Therapeutic Touch will continue to act as a credible and exemplary model to carry each therapist into her future.

In this book you will hear the voices of many TT therapists. After having traveled each summer for several decades to Therapeutic Touch camps at Camp Indralaya on Orcas Island, and to New York at Pumpkin Hollow Farm, I decided to spend all of the summer months at my beloved home and wildlife sanctuary in Columbia Falls, Montana. With the help of Pat Cole and Sandy Matheny, I sent out an invitation for TT folk to come to Montana each August for a gathering that came to be called the Therapeutic Touch Dialogues. We held our first gathering in 2010. What an adventure this turned out to be! The Dialogues birthed two studies: "'Looking Over My Shoulder,' A Study in Mindfulness" in 2012, and "Healing-at-a-Distance Exploratory Study" in 2013. I have decided to include abridged versions of these studies so that the voices of those healers can be heard by a wider audience.

My working hypothesis is that those of you who practice other disciplines of the healing arts will find that these voices resonate with your own experiences. I offer this volume to you in that spirit. It has been my life's work to study, practice, and teach Therapeutic Touch. I can say that, in my ninety-seventh year, I am confident that the future consciousness of Therapeutic Touch is in very capable hands. Ho!

COLUMBIA FALLS, MONTANA
2019

PART 1

THE WAY
OF THE HEALER

Exploring the Consciousness
of Therapeutic Touch

1

What Is Human Energy Healing?

I have been fascinated by energy healing for at least six decades. As Dora Kunz and I developed Therapeutic Touch (TT), I recognized the call to make it my lifework. The first course in healing at a university level was Frontiers in Nursing, which I initiated in 1972 as part of the New York University master's program. To date, TT has been taught at more than eighty colleges and is practiced in approximately ninety countries worldwide. Today any online search reveals a vast array of energy-healing modalities. It is clear that the realms of energy medicine have become fascinating to many throughout the world who are practicing, teaching, and researching these disciplines.

We still cannot say precisely "how" these therapies work, to the satisfaction of the Western scientific approach. However, a multitude of clinical studies have shown us that they do. This book is a synthesis of what I have observed, studied, and investigated around the world. I offer it with the hope that it will inspire others to add to the stories included here. In addition, I offer a conceptual foundation for thinking about and perhaps furthering the research on the mechanism for energy-healing effectiveness as it meets contemporary challenges to health. Since I am most familiar with TT, I use it as a model for understanding energy healing.

Therapeutic Touch has long been understood as a contemporary interpretation of several ancient healing practices that have endured through time. Ancient healing practices that are incorporated into the TT process include the laying on of hands, deep visualization, touch with and without physical contact, sustained centering of the TT therapist's consciousness, the therapist's knowledgeable use of certain of her chakras, and the intentional therapeutic use of breath and touch. Prime is the centering of the healer's consciousness; throughout the TT interaction she remains in the state of "sustained centering." This becomes the background of the process, as she includes other practices that are appropriate to the condition of each individual seeking healing.

A partner to sustained centering is the practice of compassion as power. Compassion is a benevolent positive feeling toward another, while maintaining one's equanimity and emotional detachment from the other's state of dis-ease, or energetic imbalance. Power refers to the ability to influence others. Compassion can be thought of as the catalyst or tiny chemical reaction that lights the benevolent intention to help or heal—followed by the triggering of an entire cascade of hormonal, chemical, and energetic responses in the healer to embody and then offer to the person in need.

Historically across time and cultures the healer has called upon a source of healing; any power to facilitate healing comes not *from* the healer but *through* the healer from her source. In TT the therapeutic use of the subtle energies of the universal healing field, invited by the intention of the healer, includes a sense of the ordering principles supporting the interactions of human physiology, feelings, emotions, thoughts, inspirations, and aspirations.

There is a practice we call "scaffolding," by which the centered healer offers her own healthy subtle-energy fields as a model for the healee's dysfunctional physical, psychodynamic, mental, or spiritual fields to compassionately represent for the recipient vital, healthy patterns of functioning.

Mind-to-mind communication—messages sent in silence to the patient—has been shown to provide relaxation and comfort particularly for those in critical condition, near death, or unable to communicate verbally.

Similarly, vivid visualization may arise spontaneously—what I have come to call the visualizations that come as accurate portrayals during a session—for the centered healer as she allows her intuition to receive information from the healee's field. These visualizations are often confirmed by debriefing with the healee or by subsequent events. These visions are not imagery but a kind of remote viewing of the healee's situation.

Other ancient practices include some aspects of laying on of hands, the use of breath in the expression of intentionality, and knowledgeable use of the healer's own chakra complex. These practices continue to operate efficiently in the modern world among a variety of energetic modalities, in compassionate response to a call from one in need. Which of these practices is used depends largely on the individual situation; however at a minimum these venerable therapeutic skills can integrate with one another.

The Phases of the Therapeutic Touch Process Experienced as Shifts in Consciousness

These ancient healing practices become integrated within the healing interaction to meet contemporary health challenges through the phases of the Therapeutic Touch practice.

A Call of Compassion and Centering
In the beginning it is compassion for someone in need that brings the Therapeutic Touch therapist to the healing act. Compassion as power is foundational, for it draws the therapist toward the person who is in need. Without being anchored in compassion, healing could become merely a power play of diverse vital energies used for personal interests. Compassion, of course, is a prime function of the heart chakra.

The TT therapist starts the session with a distinct shift in level of consciousness—to that of sustained centering—and she maintains that centered state throughout the session, while also employing healing techniques as needed. In this altered state of consciousness she experiences a sense of interiority embodying a stillness and a background of timelessness that can be profound. This quietude and inwardly focused attention is assumed so that the therapist can remain present to the person in need.

As Dora explained: "Centering begins with a pattern you establish within yourself. You think of your energies focused in your heart for a moment or two until you feel very still. When you have within yourself the sense of quietness—which very often is a metaphor for wholeness—then you deliberately send out the sense of caring. Once you center within yourself it is easier for you to be an instrument for healing while projecting this sense of wholeness. You gather your energies, your focus of consciousness, and just be still."[*]

Therapeutic Touch is a transpersonal process that involves a direct liaison or conscious linkage with one's Inner Self.[†] This practice occurs within a context that acknowledges the conscious recognition of alternate realities, rather than one absolute reality.

Approach
The approach can be physical or energetic; it is a reaching out to another from the impersonal space facilitated by sustained centering.

Outreach
It is at this point that the healer makes the decision to extend hands and/or energy field toward the healee. When the hands of the healer extend, she naturally holds her palms toward the healee so that her hand chakras are exposed to the subtle-energy interactions.

Search/Assessment
As the therapist becomes sensitive to these interactions, she begins to be aware of patterns in the vital-energy flows (called "cues") that become meaningful to her in reference to the healee's state of health. She begins an active search of the healee's personal fields, using her hands, her mind, and her senses. The continued search for cues in the client's fields may result in a true visualization by the healer of the client's problems,

---

[*]Dora Kunz with Dolores Krieger, Ph.D., R.N., *The Spiritual Dimension of Therapeutic Touch* (Rochester, Vt.: Bear & Company, 2004), 202.
[†]The concept of Inner Self is discussed further in chapter 3; see page 25. —*Editor*

and she begins to develop a plan for assisting those fields to become more balanced.

Rebalance and Reassessment

The plan unfolds in the next phase—rebalancing. Here the therapist helps the person seeking healing to regain a balanced state of health. Thus it is in this phase that the healing of the patient's condition may actually occur; however, it is not unusual for there to be a short time lapse or time acceleration for healing to become physically noticeable. Additionally, there may be no outward signs of "healing," particularly if what the healee needs is the feeling of relaxation and calm, of order being restored to some extent. During this phase the therapist/healer is listening closely to the field of the healee and is guided by the cues that she is picking up. The therapist often does a reassessment at this time to evaluate what changes have occurred in the fields of the healee.

Done

This final phase of the healing session describes how the TT therapist knows that she has *done* as much as she can to help the patient at that time, and she concludes the session, suggesting that the person lie down or sit quietly for ten to fifteen minutes to stabilize his now refreshed energy flow. Very frequently the healee relaxes into a short but deep nap.

Recall

A subsidiary phase, recall, notes ways the TT therapist may remember the patient and his healing session—in dream, reverie, or other subtle aspect of memory. After validating this information as well as she can— and if it is in the best interests of the patient in reference to his health— she might add this information to the data concerning their sessions. This phase was not traditionally included but became valuable in light of the focus on the TT process from the perspective of the therapist.

2

Deep Knowing through Resonance and Sentience

My interest in a conceptual framework was fostered by an early appreciation of the creative insights into the concept of human consciousness of Pierre Teilhard de Chardin (1881–1955), a French Jesuit paleontologist. His research looked back to the beginning times of living organisms on Earth and convinced him that it is primarily human consciousness that marks each of us with a singular feeling of our livingness—an awareness that we are ourselves and not another—that allows us to claim our sense of identity. Based upon his studies he concluded that promotion and development of consciousness was the primary purpose of evolution. This means that in actualizing our potential consciousness, we become more fully human.*

In his developing theory, de Chardin introduced the concept of a noosphere, which he defined as the thinking layer of Earth that he regarded as being essentially similar to the function of the Earth's biosphere, a dimension of space that surrounds Earth and contains the conditions for living. He theorized that the noosphere, created by human intelligence, has fostered conditions that now permit the extension of societal and scientific capabilities in a manner entirely different from that of any previous evolutionary stage. Essentially this implies that instead of the stimuli for human evolution coming from the environment and other events exterior

---

*Pierre Teilhard de Chardin, *The Phenomenon of Man* (New York: Harper & Row, 1975).

to the individual, human evolution will derive from its own consciousness, from—as de Chardin termed it—"the within of things." It is within this conceptualization that the future consciousness of the healer will be examined as we lay out our developing ideas of a frame of reference for the future of the transpersonal healing act.

I have long been interested in the theories of de Chardin and his ideas about human evolution as they relate to my thinking about future consciousness, so I was delighted to come across a piece by the astrophysicist and writer Adam Frank on National Public Radio in 2015:

> Right now, at this very moment, you are submerged in an invisible sea of information. Thoughts, ideas, ambitions, and instructions—they are whispering past and through you on waves of modulated electromagnetic energy. From wireless internet to satellite TV you are bathed in an endless stream of purposeful, intentional signal. And it's not just you. From the Earth's surface out to geosynchronous orbit (22,000 miles overhead), the whole planet glows with information made manifest in light (actual light, as in radio waves, microwaves, and so on). But does all that thought mean the Earth is thinking? Does that mean it's awake? Maybe it's time to consider the noosphere.*

I was intrigued to learn that there are a number of people and groups who have linked the theories of de Chardin with the World Wide Web—which a search on the internet quickly informed me.

Experiential Knowing

Other than faith or opinion, there are two major avenues to determine the authenticity of communication relative to deep healing: the logical development of theory and the projections of experiential knowing. Our present exploration is charged with the latter avenue of inquiry, experiential knowing, because fundamentally it is the healer's intention to be present to the subtle-energy flow in the fields of the healee that informs her of its moment-to-moment state. The overall focus is on the healing

---

*Adam Frank, "Can the Earth Be Conscious?" *Cosmos & Culture: Commentary on Science and Society* 13.7, National Public Radio (April 14, 2015).

process—a multilevel conscious event—as experienced by the therapist.

Reaching back to the initial stages of human communication related to healing we can imagine that gestures, guttural sounds, and body language probably preceded the word, and that the word itself was most likely articulated in an explosive expression, possibly as an early version of *ouch!* The word was likely accompanied by a manual grasping of the area that hurt, a first attempt at therapeutic touch as a reflex effort to alleviate the "owie."

The experiential descriptions of healing are remarkably consistent across eras and across diverse cultures on planet Earth. Moreover, experiential knowing is a personal awareness that stirs one deeply within. "Knowing" can be a profound understanding gained through sentience—feeling, rather than thinking—that occurs without words. Healing melds together the information that comes through sentience and through intellect into a felt sense, as the healer proceeds simultaneously on this bimodal path from "the within of things." Increasing clarity of the information from the subtle-energy streaming of the patient's field occurs for the therapist who remains present, grounded, and centered. Other potentials of higher human functions awaken, such as compassion, intuition, and, for some, a finer awareness of one's own chakra complex. The psychodynamic arc of the therapist in the throes of compassion spans sometimes incipient dimensions of silent yearnings to help or to heal those in need, and then vaults to stunning, wondrous happenings at the edge of the currently unaccountable and the frankly numinous.

Resonance as a Basis of Experiential Knowing

Resonance had its initial and most precise definition in the field of physics. When used within the context of Therapeutic Touch, this state moves us into the realm of transpersonal healing. Resonance can be seen as a demonstration of one of our early assumptions in TT: each of us is a local concentration of energy within a larger universal field.

The idea of resonance has come to have mathematical and scientific validity, as well as psychodynamic authenticity and potency. This phenomenon occurs between two identical tuning forks connected to each other by the surrounding air between them. When one tuning fork begins to vibrate, the energy carried by the sound waves through the air meets the second tuning fork. Since they are identical, they begin to vibrate at the same frequency.

Resonance also comes into play when one is pushing a child in a swing. If the pushes are synchronized with the motion of the swing—if they are in resonance—the push will enhance the swinging motion. If the pushes are irregular they cannot add energy but, rather, subtract it from the swinging motion. On the energetic level, between two people this synchronizing of frequencies can occur unintentionally; they may call this being "on the same wavelength." In Therapeutic Touch, as the healer remains centered and present to the healee the vibrational frequency of the two fields can begin to synchronize, to resonate; the healer experiences the harmony between the fields, and the patient may feel this also. The TT therapist often employs the theory of resonance when she uses the technique of scaffolding. She consciously offers the template of her own healthy and balanced field to invite the healee's field to come into resonance.

This resonant enactment occurs during the shifting of consciousness as the therapist probes the healing partner's* subtle-energy fields during the TT search. As the therapist locates subtle-energy patterns that are out of balance, her own energy, attitudes, and values shift in compassionate response through the deeper ranges of sympathy, identity, empathy, and synchronization, culminating in compassion as power.

David Spangler, a world-renowned psychic investigator who is unusually gifted, gives us a hint of how resonance can be used psychodynamically when he states, "Travel on the inner [his term for the domain of subtle energies] is through resonance, relationships, and connections."†

For a number of years Spangler had a relationship with a nonphysical teacher named John. He describes their way of communication:

---

*The healer and healee—the person seeking healing—work together in partnership to investigate and attempt to resolve the issue. They are thus considered to be healing partners. In this book the term "healing partner" is used interchangeably with patient/client/recipient/healee. —*Editor*
†David Spangler, *Apprenticed to Spirit: The Education of a Soul* (New York: Penguin Group, 2011), 125.

Trying to "talk" to me in a conventional way was both too slow and too limited for the communication we needed. Communion became the basis for communication between us, and this required a high degree of energy synchronization, configuration, and resonance. John didn't just tell me about something; he drew me into the experience of it so that I could see it through his eyes. . . . [We] established a basic resonance together, like tying an energy string between us so that we were connected.*

In TT practice, resonance is most intimately related to the constant change of energetic flow. In its basic sense resonance is concerned with harmonic relations; dissonance concerns itself with sources of disharmony. The therapist experientially senses the energetic flows variously as waves, rhythm, particles, and other nonphysical perceptions, such as vibration, oscillation, reverberation, echo, or other subtle-energy patterns.

Resonance is built into our DNA. The easiest access to resonance is through the heart chakra. The initial vibration that the gestating child experiences is the vibration of the mother's heartbeat. The heart chakra apparently translates feelings and beliefs into electrical and magnetic waves, as well as vibration. In this way the pregnant mother communes with her child through her heartbeats.

Resonance in the context of healing provides the milieu, the atmosphere, the background, the setting, the surround. Resonance between healer and healee invites those in need to "bounce back," to resound in harmony, integration, and balance.

To understand the phenomenon of resonance, it is important to acknowledge that the open space—like that between the tuning forks—is not empty. An individual's space extends in distances exceeding ten feet, depending on its state of intensity (as confirmed by bioelectrical measurement). Transpersonal healing, which is multidimensional, happens within this domain. The living fields are permeated with intent, aspirations, and meaning that go beyond faith, belief, and cultural mores. There is information in the open space that can be communicated mind-to-mind and heart-to-heart.

---

*David Spangler, *Apprenticed to Spirit*, 74 and 98.

The mathematician Arthur Eddington describes the experience of healing interactions in the open space: "We used to think that if we knew one, we knew two, because one and one are two. We are finding that we must learn a great deal more about *and.*"* When teaching a beginning class in Therapeutic Touch, one of the very early exercises we introduce to students is extending hands out in front of themselves with palms facing each other. We direct that people move their palms toward each other and then farther apart, slowly moving the hands back and forth, separating them and bringing them back together. Most people have the experience of some kind of energetic sensation between their moving palms. This demonstrates that the open space is not empty, which allows the understanding that between the two hands (one and one) we are experiencing the "*and.*" This exercise is also taught in other modes of energy healing.

Deep Knowing during Healing

Several factors begin to impress themselves onto a consideration of a conceptual framework of Therapeutic Touch as transpersonal healing:

- Experiential knowing through sentience is the "native language" of transpersonal healing. Communing mind-to-mind is a natural method of exchanging information, transmitting relationships, or sensing deep emotions. Sentience is the power of perception by the senses, rather than by structured logic, to understand one's inner world more clearly. Deep sentience has a powerful, subtle effect on the limbic system.
- Compassion is the entry point into the process of healing. It is a highly human function. The term "compassion" has Latin roots: *com* means with, and *pati* means to bear or to suffer with a person who is in anguish or going through a difficult ordeal. Intense compassion profoundly stimulates the psyche, which assists the healer on her journey as she seeks out or clarifies relationships with her Inner Self. Compassion demands keen discrimination and a willingness to feel with the patient while staying detached. It is a

---

*Alan L. Mackay, *A Dictionary of Scientific Quotations* (Abingdon, UK: CRC Press, 1991), 79.

complex state. The centered therapist needs to have her own solid base of emotional experiences in order to recognize that the healing partner is having difficulties, is suffering, or is experiencing limited functions, and that *these difficulties are not her own.*

- When sensing the misery and suffering of the one in need, the therapist may become aware of deep pain, anguish, and hurt. I believe these perceptions are evoked from the depths of her limbic system. Although the limbic system is not fully understood at this time, it is known that some of our profound emotions are connected to it. It has been shown that emotions can involve deep brain structures: the amygdala, hippocampus, thalamus, and olfactory lobe. By staying centered and connected, the therapist may be able to assist in the rebalancing of these emotions within the healee—without the need to be consciously aware of them.

As noted, at the same time that the therapist is in the throes of compassion for the suffering and disorder of the patient, a compelling force is called up from within her being. At first, during—or even before—the approach phase she may begin to be aware of "differences," vague and ambiguous sensations that with increased attention or focus may "gel" or cohere as the therapist identifies them as cues. Even during the approach, she finds herself engaged in an act of subtle exploration. With sentience as ally, her senses become a major avenue for "getting

Major Components of the Limbic System

Deep emotions and spirituality may be rooted in, or connected to, the amygdala, the hippocampus, the thalamus, and the olfactory lobe.

in touch with" the healing partner's subtle-energy fields. The therapist sharpens her perception of the cues as she shifts her consciousness to the search/assessment phase of the healing process.

Sentience is relied on as the therapist literally "feels" her way and experiences increased clarity in reference to the cues she is picking up from the healing partner's vital-energy field. During this intense time a ray of intuition may flash to illuminate the therapist's understanding of how she might help the patient. Deeply engaged in the search, the therapist can actually feel herself "reach" for the subtle-energy fields of the person in need. This is an expression of sentience, the lived experience of the search phase. In practice we have found that the energies of pain, fatigue, and anxiety may be the easiest to differentiate among the irregularities and imbalances in the patient's fields.

As the process unfolds and transforms itself as transpersonal healing, the inner journey of the therapist brings her into a more lucid relationship with the guidance of her Inner Self. A clear word-for-word translation of that experience has been challenging.

Let us attempt to give this "effortless effort" of transpersonal healing a translation from the realm of experiential knowing through sentience. Although it is not always easy to put into words, following are some changes that have been observed within the person in the role of healer during actual sessions and in other aspects of her life:

- Effortlessly, the therapist enters a sustained centered state of consciousness, which she maintains until the end of the healing session.
- As a deep relaxation response is experienced by the patient, a decided shift in consciousness is felt by the therapist herself. One quality of this is a deepening quietude; a stillness enfolds the healing milieu.
- In this sensitive seeking-the-within mode, the therapist consciously uses her vital-energy field and possibly her chakra complex to reach out to the other.
- Then the therapist may go "inth" (that is, she focuses her attention significantly more than she would during simple everyday activities, transcending the usual physical dimensions of length, width, and breadth).
- Once she identifies the areas of imbalance in the healing partner's

fields, the therapist assesses their qualities to better understand the meaning of the cues she is receiving. Her focus of attention sharpens.

- She resorts to metaphors or invents terms to communicate the inexpressible or nonlinguistic experiences she is undergoing.

- Using her hands in this context engages the hand chakras, which have strong, though subtle, relationships with the heart chakra. This allows deeper insight and keener discernment, and her mind now easily picks up hints as she assesses the cues in the fields of the patient.

- As the session continues, the subtle-energy interactions between healer and healee create a transpersonal medium that facilitates an understanding of the patterning of cues the therapist perceives in the patient's field.

- The therapist's personal fields are being prepared by compassion to reflect an increasingly profound healing atmosphere. According to the theories of de Chardin, her relationship to the noosphere is being stabilized.

- Meanwhile, the fine-energy dynamics of this interchange occur at deep levels of the therapist's consciousness, creating an atmosphere that strongly resembles that of a moving meditative state. She is becoming a clearer, more highly tuned instrument of healing.

Over the years, some of the following changes have been observed among TT therapists in their daily lives:

- The therapist becomes more aware of her personal identification with her Inner Self, beginning to be aware of her "within" at times other than during the TT interactions.

- As Inner Self becomes actively involved in her daily life, she reciprocally seeks out her path, her inner journey, in her role as healer. Her self-search now significantly intensifies, and her realization of the role she is playing becomes more personally meaningful. It "lights up"—that is, it illumines her being.

- In her healing practice she may begin to note a greater degree of sensitivity to, and an increase in, the conscious use of her chakras, an ancient way of self-awakening that gives her valid access to the realm of deeper knowing.

- There is strong possibility for a decided increase in the acuity of her perceptions. For instance, particularly during the search phase, a deep knowing beyond everyday cognition rises to consciousness. As she may sense a true mind-to-mind connection with the patient, the therapist enters communication at the transpersonal level of consciousness. When not engaged in the healing sessions, she may begin to notice that she is increasingly relying on her intuition in day-to-day interactions.

- Relying more on her intuition as she begins to test it out and understand its ways, she confidently entertains intimations of next steps that will enforce and fortify her sensitivity and her competency.

- The therapist may become aware of profound psychodynamic, mental, and spiritual changes that reflect positively in her now-sharpened ability to compassionately help those in need. This reflection is mirrored in behavior, thought, and meditations as she continues to experience the fine nuances of her inner journey.

During a TT session, over and over, the therapist experiences the shift between the "within" of her Inner Self and the "without" of the needs of the healee in front of her. The shifting effects of compassionate focus during TT are depicted in the following chart.

Effect on the Process (Deepening Insight into TT Process)	Effect on the Therapist (Deepening Insight into Self)
Sustained centering	Emergence of Inner Self
Healing as a moving meditation	Stillness and timelessness
Entry point to multiple realities	Sense of confidence
Actualization of potentialities	In-depth exploration of Inner Self
Multifield integration	Potentiation of the chakras
Mind-to-mind search and rebalance	Compassion as power
Unfolding of intuition	Explicit intentionality
Outflow of creativity	Vivid visualization

3

The Story of David's Healing

Each person's path is, of course, individually organized and personally configured. Below is an account as experienced in a recent Therapeutic Touch healing interaction, a skilled engagement between an intelligent, courageous, and trusting healing partner (healee) who had been injured, a concerned allopathic medical team, a loving spouse who happened to be an experienced and talented massage therapist and herbalist, and a mature and knowledgeable Therapeutic Touch therapist (the author).

The healing sessions were conducted outdoors in full sunlight on dedicated land with a mountain nearby, all of which freely contributed their unique energies. Also adding to this natural healing environment was Kate, the family guard dog, and four horses who roamed freely on the lawn, occasionally wandering up to insert themselves directly into the session with the healing partner, with whom they obviously had a strong bond.

The incident that precipitated this scenario occurred when David, a friend and neighbor who became the healing partner in this story, helped a neighbor at a nearby ranch with the late spring round-up and transportation of free-range cows that had been left to overwinter on nearby land. Under usual circumstances the cows would have been taken to a corral on the ranch for about two weeks to get accustomed to having humans and horses about them, and also to being restricted within the corral. However, in this case it had been decided to proceed directly to the branding stage.

Astride his horse Archie, David separated out a cow to bring in and lassoed her, at which point the cow, accustomed to the freedom of living on the range, went berserk. David let go of the lariat, as was appropriate. However, the end of the lariat whipped around, catching on the saddle and repeatedly wrapping itself around Archie's legs, jerking the horse's legs out from under him. When Archie went down, he pinned David under his 1,350-pound body.

Archie's subsequent actions were only one of several miracles that day, for he lay quietly, only turning his head toward David to see where he was lying. Had he moved he might have added to David's injuries. Another unusual happening was that a woman working the nearby bushes saw David go down. She rushed to him and, despite weighing only about 110 pounds, managed to drag him out from under his horse. At the perfect moment Archie shifted his hindquarters so that David could be removed. Still another remarkable bit of synchronicity occurred: at the time of the accident an emergency vehicle was driving past the ranch and was hailed, enabling David to be rapidly transported to the hospital.

Emergency measures were initiated en route, and David was fully examined upon arrival. Major findings were:

- Sixteen ribs were fractured, puncturing one of his lungs.
- A clavicle was broken.
- The right shoulder was crushed.
- His right wrist was broken.
- There were numerous hematomas and several small cuts.
- The spleen was lacerated.
- He was conscious, but obviously in shock.

The Therapeutic Touch Frame of Reference

David is an independent farrier who works the ranches of Northwest Montana; he is lean and normally healthy. He was discharged from the hospital after a few days, with a follow-up visit scheduled. He phoned me upon returning home and I treated him with Therapeutic Touch at his home every weekday for the next three weeks, and did healing at-a-distance on the weekends.

Therapeutic Touch is a transpersonal process that involves a direct liaison or conscious linkage with the Inner Self. This practice occurs within a context that acknowledges the conscious recognition of alternate realities, rather than one absolute reality.

The concept of Inner Self is one that held special meaning for Dora Kunz in relation to Therapeutic Touch. She explained it this way: "Each of us has a sense of peace and quiet within. Although we are not usually aware of it, I believe that this sense characterizes an aspect of what I call the 'Inner Self.' Many people call it 'soul.' I use the term Inner Self because it has no other connotations; it has not been defined." She explained that this Inner Self has many aspects.

> One aspect—perhaps the most significant—is a sense of basic unity at the deepest level we can reach. This is the feeling that we are all bound closely together, a sense of genuine brotherhood. In addition to the seeds of peace and quiet within, the Inner Self has several levels of consciousness. At the highest level of that consciousness we are all bound together in an orderly process. We all have these different levels of consciousness, which give us access to the many aspects of the Inner Self.*

In Therapeutic Touch practice, the Inner Self can be relied on to support the state of sustained centering; and this aspect of ourselves is often used to reach out to the recipient during the session. As Dora told us: "During a healing you can acknowledge your Inner Self and then send the patient energy at that more subtle level. There is this recognition by the healee of *Here is someone who knows that I am that Inner Self and who understands what I am going through.†*

Within the realms of healing there are many ways—as many,

---

*Dora Kunz with Dolores Krieger, *The Spiritual Dimension of Therapeutic Touch* (Rochester, Vt.: Bear & Company, 2004), 199.
†Dora Kunz with Dolores Krieger, *The Spiritual Dimension of Therapeutic Touch,* 199–200.

perhaps, as there are ways for people to relate to one another. What does Therapeutic Touch offer that is unique? It is that the quest of the TT therapist is one of self-realization in conscious liaison with her Inner Self, while engaged in compassionate outreach to those who are ill, in trauma, or whose life systems are otherwise out of balance. She sets the stage for this intimate therapeutic interaction as she goes into the state of consciousness known as "sustained centering" at the beginning of the TT session and, in an act of interiority, seeks her personal relationship with her Inner Self. It is the maintenance of the state of sustained centering that provides an appropriate milieu for her Inner Self so that this state of beingness can actively enter into and support her efforts during the healing interaction.

The TT therapist assesses the healing partner's subtle-energy fields, sensing the cues she is picking up; the aha! moment culminates, and she comes to realize the therapeutic maneuvers she should employ to repattern and rebalance her healing partner's subtle-energy fields. It is now—as she acknowledges this realization and engages the appropriate forces tethered to her intentionality to modulate, shift, or direct the healing partner's pranic flow for his therapeutic well-being—that the healing moment is potentiated.

Facilitating David's Therapeutic Touch Process

As a TT therapist I would expedite this for David in at least one of four ways noted below, or in a mix-and-match of them as needed.

1. I would begin by centering and making myself aware of natural, undifferentiated healing energies that had gathered around my wounded healing partner; that is, I would become a conduit for the universal healing field, allowing the now focused healing energies to flow through my healthy self to my healing partner, David.
2. Through the resolute and willful use of my intentionality, I would focus available subtle energies from my solar plexus chakra to my heart chakra, and then through David's heart chakra. As needed I would go more deeply, doing a "Deep Dee," focusing my attention

deeply within to get a sense of my own chakra complex, beginning at the lowermost or most dense, and then I'd successively give my attention to those upper chakras that have a finer flow. At each successive level of consciousness I would test my sense of my healing partner's corresponding chakras; that is, in an ascending manner I would compare my sense of each of the chakras of my own complex, which I know very well, to the similar chakra in my healing partner's complex.

3. If I sensed a sympathetic reaction, a resonance between our chakras, I would assume his chakra was in a conscious, aware, functioning state, as was mine. If my sense of his chakra was one of dissonance, I'd assume his was not functioning as well as mine and I would keep my focus on the level of consciousness we shared and do my inner therapeutic work from there. Later I would continue to sensitively probe further into the flow of the finer energies of his chakra complex until I no longer felt the dissonance.

4. Working through my heart chakra, I would continue to offer myself as a conduit for the universal healing field. Meanwhile (it is possible to think of more than one thing at a time) I would try to clearly visualize my connection to the healing partner's Inner Self. Once I had stabilized this perception, I would focus this visualization through the lens of my crown chakra, and then, working with my Inner Self, whose signs of presence are unmistakable to me, I would continue to support David.

A Spectrum of Reliable Expectations

As a result of extensive research and responsible observation, there are several reliable expectations that I could anticipate from my Therapeutic Touch sessions with David:

1. I could expect that David would exhibit a deep relaxation response within the first two to four minutes of the TT session; that is, there would be a significant reduction in his blood pressure and pulse rate. In addition, there would be an increased dilation of the

vessels of his peripheral vascular system, which would be observable by a generalized pinking—a slight flushing of his skin early in the TT session.

2. There would be a reduction in pain level and, from previous research cited elsewhere, we also know that there could be an accompanying decrease in uses of analgesics and an enhancement of their effect on him.

3. TT would promote an emotional response, which would act to increase the general effectiveness of symptom management.

4. The healing process itself could accelerate, both physically and psychodynamically.

5. Because of this cumulative effect of the TT process, the impact of post-trauma shock would be considerably dampened. There could be decreased anxiety and a lessening of symptoms as follows:

- Relief of nausea
- Enhancement of breathing
- Reduction in level of irritability

On the other hand, I also realized that there were several factors that might importantly delimit the extent to which healing could take place. Notably these might include:

- The destiny of this healing partner, a mysterious notion that has been given substantial credence in this Newer Age. (See the third major assumption in chapter 5 for discussion of the influence of one's destiny on the healing process.)
- The healing partner's willingness to engage himself in his own healing process; that is, to be accepting of the therapeutic intervention and allowing it to happen in its own way.
- The healing partner's ability to relax and permit others to help him to relax, so that the healing process itself could most easily and smoothly permeate the body.
- And—particularly in the case of an active and independent person such as David—his decision to return to full activity before the healing process had made significant progress.

Considerations and Cautions Regarding the Healer's Intervention in This Instance

For David's sake as well as my own, it was important for me to be mindful of subtle as well as gross effects of my healing intervention. These perceptions included:

- Appreciation of the possibility of a too-intense identification with the suffering of my healing partner.
- Recognition of a wavering of my own sense of self, and a projection of David's problems onto myself.
- Opening the gates to possibilities of psychological transference and countertransference.
- Fostering feelings that might arise in David re dependence on myself.

There are several safeguards built into the Therapeutic Touch model against such occurrences. For instance:

- It is imperative to remain calm, through sustained centering, during the healing session, and emotionally detached from the results of the interaction. "The outcome is not in our hands," as Dora Kunz often reminded us.
- Equally essential is the therapist's maintenance of a sense of harmony and singleness of purpose with her Inner Self.
- It is important to keep uppermost in mind a compassionate awareness of the physical suffering and psychological needs of the healee.
- It is important to gently enfold the healing partner with a sense of intentionality that is oriented to the needs of his greatest good.

Additionally, in view of the significance of personal motivations in offering my healing abilities, it was also very important that I try to understand and acknowledge to myself why I was engaged in this healing interaction. Was it simply because David was a friend who asked for help that I was able to give him, or was it to show off my healing abilities to neighbors? Was my involvement based in a true outflow of compassion, or was it instigated in the service of my ego? Finally, of course: If I have to ask the question, what does the question itself say about the questioner?

How I Worked the Therapeutic Touch Process

I first saw David on the eighth day after the accident. I was aware almost immediately that, understandably, he still suffered from the aftermath of the shock, and this was augmented by fear about the condition in which he now found himself and by anxiety and uncertainty about his future. I deeply centered myself as I approached him, and after a short talk about details of his accident and how I might help him, I set about stabilizing his vital signs, including the considerable pain he was experiencing. As a relaxation response began to set in, I shifted my focus slightly to deal further with the deeper reaches of the pain, stress, and utter fatigue that still gripped him. I saw a generalized flush tinge his skin and realized that the relaxation response had deepened. I slowly began to deal with the psychological reality of his accident by shifting into Deep Dee to help him with his still vivid thoughts, feelings, and memories about the accident.

As previously noted, I worked on-site for three weeks, for about one hour on each weekday, and I did healing at-a-distance on weekends. In addition to the TT maneuvers noted above, I knew I could depend on various natural functions of the universal healing field, such as an intrinsic order and intelligence that is evoked by compassion and can be consciously reinforced by the TT therapist. David's wife, Helen, was in attendance frequently, and her positive and sensitive presence was loving and reassuring and gave the sessions a focus that was of considerable help.

We have come to understand that Therapeutic Touch may include communion with genres of intelligences other than those ordinarily perceived, such as angelic presences. Working with David during his healing, I connected with the natural energies that were in abundance on this responsive land: the strong presence of the nearby mountain and the curious animals, Archie among them, who watched with a gentle but alert eye for David's safety. All shared their powerful, personal emanations of living energies. It was interesting to me to sense that whereas Katie, the dog, seemed to send unconditional love, particularly to David, the sense I got from the keenly alert horses was the projection of a kind of organizing power, which I felt to be very helpful in directing the flow of prana—vital energy—to him.

In all this multitiered interaction I "listened" deeply to the cues as they arose to my perception. One day while so engaged I became aware of a new (to me) subtle energy deep in David's solar plexus that extended to his throat chakra. It seemed to be related to his fear, which still lingered, and so I worked with that, too. To my delight, that night while reading a neurology textbook I had just received, I happened upon a description of neural connections in exactly the area I had come across while working with him earlier in that day. (Not exactly a confirmation of chakra function, but it was close, wasn't it?)

What I Was Hoping to Find

What were the touchstones I was seeking in these TT healing sessions? Primarily I was checking and rechecking for nonphysical signs of subtle-energy balance, symmetry, and the subtle rush of pranic streaming, or flow.* After evaluating these signs I went on to sense cues indicative of intensity. For instance, the sense of congestion indicates to me where my healing partner's pain is being felt by him. In my personal vocabulary of energetic cues, it makes itself known by a feeling similar to a weak electric shock. Perceived as a tingling sensation in my hand chakras, these little shocks give me a clue to areas of subtle-energy deficit that are felt as pain. In the healing partner's vital-energy field I pick up sensations that I experience in my personal vocabulary of energetic perceptions as a hot–cold spectrum of temperature, to locate concentrations of infection and/or inflammation. In my experience, felt disturbances in the underlying rhythm of the pranic flow may indicate that there is a problem in the endocrine glands or the chakras.

I have also found that a sense of pressure may indicate a problem with the circulatory system. At times I have found that high blood pressure may be perceived in the vital-energy field overlying the internal

---

*Dolores Krieger is describing the process of Therapeutic Touch as she came to understand the dynamics from the perspective of the chakra system. This analysis came to her over her many years immersed in the practice, study, and research of TT. Please note that it is not necessary to hold this perspective in the conscious mind to learn and practice Therapeutic Touch. —*Editor*

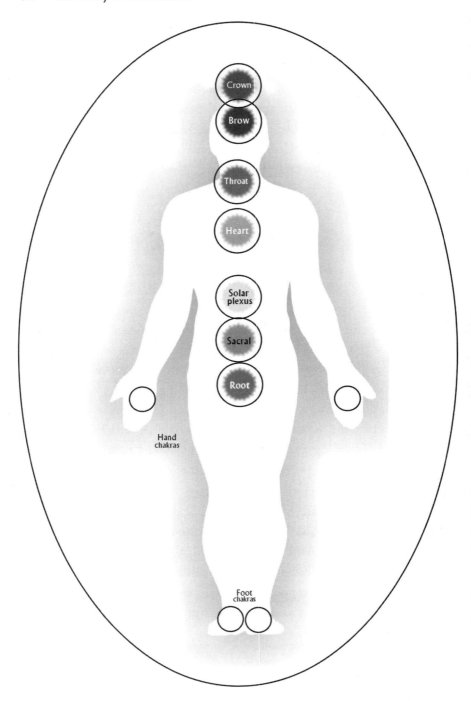

Chakras are understood to be centers of energy and consciousness in the subtle body.

carotid vessels. A slightly different perception of compression may indicate the presence of a blood clot in the system. These are interpretations of perceptions that I have tested out many times, so as to avoid impulse, fantasy, exaggeration, or wishful thinking—the Four Dragons of TT.

I used all these strategies singly or in combination, and often tinged them (visualized in my mind) with a sense of an appropriate color (or colors, for I find it is possible to hold in my mind combinations of colors simultaneously). The colors that I projected to my healing partner I perceived as being interspersed with tiny, vivid glitters or glints of intense blue-silver or yellow-gold, whichever was appropriate to the situation. When projecting and directing energy to the healing partner, and through his field, the unwavering intention was that this energy emerged from the universal healing field, through me as an "instrument of healing," as Dora would often remind us, and continued to move *through* (not just to) the field of the partner.

I relied upon the stream of information available during the days that followed, particularly staying mindful of the emotional trauma connected with the accident. In addition, I searched David's pelvic area several times for signs of internal bleeding, clots, or difficulty with blood circulation, or for indications of cracks or additional bone fractures. I tried to be sensitive to changes in subtle-energy flows, particularly as I worked over his spleen, and I also checked "behind" the lower reaches of his ribcage. Frequently I tried to go in depth (inth) around his upper cervical area, seeking out subtle signs of imbalances in the field around the spinal cord, and lower in the spinal column for cues of other trauma that might have escaped initial observation. In particular, I tried to keep sensitive to any indications of change in the level of emotional components, such as unresolved pockets of fear and anxiety.

After the second week of treatment, David kept his appointment with his medical doctor who, after examining him said, "You are doing so much better than we expected!" We continued the Therapeutic Touch healing sessions for a third week, until I had to leave town to fulfill prior engagements. I returned two weeks later to find that David, although looking quite fatigued, was now working part-time and fulfilling his daily activities.

4

Energy Healing as a Humanization of Energy

Energy healing involves the intangible but very real energy surrounding and interpenetrating all living things to address imbalances within a human energy field, both the visible, physical system of the body and the invisible, energetic system.

Patterns of Vital-Energy Flow

It is the fundamental patterning and repatterning of the nonphysical subtle-energy (pranic) flows of the vital-energy, psychodynamic, and conceptual fields that are the basis for what we know as physical functions, behavioral patterns, networks of feelings and drives, thoughts, and intuitions. These constellations are encoded in the individual's pranic streaming and are known as that person's distinctive characteristics. The healer perceives these flows in a variety of ways, including but not limited to:

- Breaks in subtle-energy flow, a sense of vital-energy deficit or vital-energy hyperactivity, an indication of pressure or fullness, signs of congestion or sluggishness in the vital-energy flow, or blockages that restrict that streaming.
- Differences in flow in the field on the right and left sides of the recipient's body.

- Metaphoric descriptions of energetic sensations such as temperature differentials of heat or cold, a sense of tingling, or slight electric shock. Over time each healer typically develops her own personal vocabulary of metaphors to describe the ineffable nature of the patterns of energy flows.
- Rare moments of intuition and true insight, sensing a thought or emotion held by the healee.

As these patterns of vital energy flow through the healer's hand chakras, they are given meaning in her mind. The information she picks up from the cues can be explicit, so that not only can the therapist locate the cue in the healee's vital-energy field, she also may get a sense of qualitative factors. For example, she might discern:

- Whether the healee's problem can be treated most efficiently by Therapeutic Touch
- The intensity of the condition
- Whether the cue represents an old vital-energy scar or a recent problem

With increased ability the TT therapist's assessment of the problem (the search) can become more finely attuned. For example, not only can she locate where the problem is but under some conditions the therapist also can get a sense of whether it is related to other cues, and in a moment of vivid visualization she might be able to perceive the circumstances surrounding its origin.

Several additional ancient healing practices mentioned previously also contribute to the "glue" that holds the Therapeutic Touch healing process together:

Sustained centering pervades all healing action in Therapeutic Touch, from the onset of the intention to help or heal through the end of the session. It also critically supports the unitary engagement of the therapist with the universal healing field.

Concentration as focused attention offers space, which can provide a point of convergence for the power of intentionality.

Visualization from the state of sustained centering is one of the ways the healer receives information about the quality of flow in the healee's energy fields. The information may come as visual metaphors indicating the healee's state of health and quality of life, and sometimes origins of his illness. This is often a way that the healer receives information when the healee is in a different location.

Mind-to-mind communication can play a role in the practice of techniques particularly for someone who is dying, has organic brain damage, is emotionally unstable, or is experiencing other crises.

Integration is crucial to handling complex emotional situations that present themselves to the therapist. As she remains sensitive to these situations, she may also become aware of information that could be at the core of an individual's illness. The process of integration is supported in the healer during periods when she is immersed in stillness and inner quietude, and in moments of realization of the unitive nature of all that is living.

Fundamental Agencies of Consciousness

Many of these experiences occur in a nonphysical realm and translate poorly into spoken language. How, then, does the healer communicate to others her own personal experience of the healing process as it takes place between herself and the healing partner? A partial answer is that the experience makes itself known to the therapist through fundamental agencies of consciousness, such as attention, intuition, and memory. During the TT session the therapist often becomes aware of emotions in the healee's field; this is a time that sustained centering is critical in the ability of the therapist to remain detached and simply observe without taking on the emotion of the other. Mind-to-mind communication is a reliable strategy often used by healers. In the silence of the healing milieu the therapist connects with her Inner Self and "talks" to the healee, sending messages of understanding and support. In this silence a response may come from the field or the Inner Self of the healee.

Clairvoyance and precognition are abilities that therapists may come to experience as facets of the development of their natural potential for healing (as stated in the first major assumption, see chapter 5). Clairvoyance—clear seeing—is the ability to perceive matters beyond the range of ordinary perception. An example of this came in a TT session in which the healer sensed the presence of a black dog. The therapist recalls, "During the treatment this large black dog kept popping into my awareness, first sitting behind her, and then closer to her lap. At one point I fully opened my eyes, as I wasn't sure there wasn't a physical dog in the room; that's how dominant the presence was. So I asked her if she had any connection to a large black dog. She gasped and said incredulously, 'How did you know that?' Tears began. Apparently she had a very special relationship with this large black dog." This is a wonderful example of how information comes from a healee's field. This is also an example of vivid visualization.

Precognition, an aspect of clairvoyance, is defined as the knowledge or prediction of future events without the possibility of influence from present evidence. One healer tells the story of her experience through hospice, with a woman in the end stage of Parkinson's. Her body was completely bound up and she had lost the ability to speak. After several weekly sessions the TT therapist had a feeling one day that the patient was preparing for her death. Knowing that this woman was quite special to the hospice volunteer coordinator, the TT volunteer called hospice to report this sense she had, in case the coordinator would want to visit the patient. The volunteer received a call back later that day to reassure her that the patient had been medically checked and that her condition was unchanged. Two days later, hospice called the volunteer again to report that the patient had died. And "How did you know?" was the question. This experience has been repeated numerous times over the years by those who have had TT interactions with those near the end of life.

Synesthesia is the condition in which one sense is simultaneously perceived by one or more additional senses. Carolyn Hart, an artist and author, has experienced synesthesia since childhood. She writes, "I have color-tactile synesthesia; I feel colors inside my mouth, not as flavors but as tactile experiences such as cold, hot, coarse, soft, or bumpy." Here is another aspect of what Carolyn experiences: "I also have synesthesia for pain; I get stinging electrical pain that shoots down my sacral dermatomes* when I see another person's wounds or injuries. Like all of my synesthesias, this experience has been with me my entire life. When I was about three years old, I remember going to the market with my mother and my older sister, who was five years old or so. The market had a heavy, swinging door that could be opened with either a push or a pull. My sister tried to push the door open but she wasn't strong enough. The door swung closed on her finger, ripping off her fingernail. As blood dripped down her hand, I felt a sizzling electrical pain shoot down my legs, from my hips to my heels. It was very painful and came in quick flashes."

People who are drawn to the healing arts are very often already sensitive in a variety of ways, easily feel empathy for others' suffering, and may be familiar with these kinds of sensations. It is the state of consciousness of sustained centering that protects the individual in the role of healer from becoming personally affected, physically or energetically, by the physical symptoms, emotions, and thoughts of the person in need.

Then, thrown back upon her perceptions of the field of the healing partner—seeking to describe the cues coming from the field in order to make her experiences understandable to others—the TT therapist calls upon figures of speech, such as metaphor, analogy, and symbol. The following are some of the terms commonly used by the therapist to describe what the cues "feel like":

- Heat/cold
- Little electric shocks
- Pressure variations
- Ruffles
- Bubbles
- Congestion/blocks
- Changes in color
- Waves
- Intuitive visualizations
- Tingling

---

*A dermatome is an area of skin that is supplied by a single spinal nerve. These nerves relay sensory, motor, and autonomic information between the body and the brain or central nervous system. —*Editor*

A fair question would be: Do these terms adequately convey meaning at a pragmatic, physical level?

With little exception I think the answer is yes—if one is willing to accept a bit of creative imagination. As well, communication about the healing process can define itself as a conscious act. Over the years I have been drawn back to a taxonomy of discrete and distinct paranormal states of consciousness developed by Charles T. Tart in his classic, *States of Consciousness*.* With a deep bow of gratitude to Dr. Tart, one of the founders of transpersonal psychology, I submit my free interpretation of nine of his criteria.

Hypothesis: the Therapeutic Touch therapist experiences a clear awareness of nine of Tart's taxonomy of specific states of consciousness during engagement with the Therapeutic Touch process. We further hypothesize that those practicing other forms of healing experience some or all of these states of consciousness.

Tart's Taxonomy in Reference to Healing

Self-awareness. During the session the therapist is discerning and responsive to physical and subtle levels of sensibility.

Sensation. The therapist perceives subtle-energy sensations through the hands, mind, or intuition, which she verbalizes as cues. This occurs during the Therapeutic Touch assessment phase.

Emotion. She may perceive cues that express variations in emotional energy during the search phase of TT, which the experienced TT therapist may associate with the heart, throat, and solar plexus chakras.

Empathy. While she discerns emotional imbalances in the client, she remains emotionally detached as she differentiates these energetic variations from her personal self.

Unition. The therapist experiences a sense of timelessness and unity during the healing session while she maintains the state of sustained centering.

*Charles T. Tart, Ph.D., *States of Consciousness* (Lincoln, Neb.: iUniverse.com, Inc., 2000), 12–13.

Intuition. As the therapist increases her sensitivity to her Inner Self she often experiences flashes of useful insight.

Healing. During the rebalancing phase, the therapist facilitates the return of energetic (pranic) healing balance and order to dysfunctional subtle energy flows. She discerns changes in the patterns of subtle-energy exhibited by the recipient, most often through her hands or intuition.

Completion. She accomplishes this during the reassessment phase when she rechecks the client for details and compares this against memory of how subtle cues may often present when in a state of order.

Memory. She may revisit the session in reverie or dreams and, if relevant, add this new information to notes on the process.

It should be noted that the reason a taxonomy—such as has been worked out above for the Therapeutic Touch process—is valuable is because it essentially defines the classification system of a body of thought. The logic upon which that system is based is implicit in the classification. A taxonomy of Therapeutic Touch speaks to the authority, credibility, and authenticity of how the experience of that person playing the role of healer is communicated to others by specifying the significant words describing that inner experience.

The point to be made, however, is this: At present, both in Therapeutic Touch and across a variety of healing modalities, the healer has at her command a few terms that convey her experiences during the healing act. These terms are typically impressionistic and can only partially translate the actual fullness and authenticity of pivotal transpersonal experiences of the healing interaction. One consequence is that the TT therapist and others who practice related modes of healing often fail to meet formal requirements of Western research and teaching. Anecdotal experience of the healing act is often discounted by conventional Western researchers and educators, since both of these disciplines base their standards for verification of valid content of Western thought on clear replication of claimed states of consciousness.

The current work on the taxonomy of Therapeutic Touch is but a beginning exploration of the range of significant, often subtle, experiences that are evoked during a healing session by the call of compassion to help or to heal those in need. Definitive clarity of the therapist's experience during the healing act would support the necessary formal recognition of energetic healing modalities.

Search for the Inner Self

It should be remembered that the Therapeutic Touch process is a contemporary interpretation of several ancient healing practices that are concerned with the knowledgeable use of the therapeutic functions of the human energy field. Within that context, TT is a conscious act (as we see from its adherence to Tart's taxonomy) that is based upon a body of knowledge derived from:

- Deep experiential knowledge that grows over time into a personal knowing
- Tested insights about the Therapeutic Touch healing process
- Logical deduction, formal and clinical research findings
- A compendium of world literature concerning the therapeutic use of vital human energies

As portrayed within the mature experience of the Therapeutic Touch healing process, TT invites the conscious, full engagement of the healer's own access to vital-energy flow in the compassionate interest of helping another person. Healing through the use of the Therapeutic Touch process—and other modes of energy healing—can then be thought of as a humanization of energies offered with this intention.

It is in the process of humanizing vital energy and making it one's own that the healer begins to work seriously toward potentiating previously dormant, often unrealized abilities within herself to assist in the compassionate interest of supporting another person who is energetically or physically in a state of imbalance. As this occurs again and again with TT healers, we observe a living demonstration of the first major assumption: healing is a natural human potential.

As we have seen, the healer is profoundly motivated by compassion, from which state of consciousness she projects a sense of order toward the consenting healee who is in need and often pressed by necessities and urgencies of a critical nature. This arena of heightened human interaction lends an atmosphere of spiritual tension to the dynamism, which links this therapeutic network and impresses itself upon the sensitive healer. Meanwhile the healer is acting as a conduit for the restorative forces of the universal healing field to support the healee's ill, weakened, or traumatized energy systems. The healer maintains a state of interiority during the healing interaction as her yearning to help or to heal leads her to seek within for her own deep-seated connection to the universal field. First as a hint, but then as an increasing reality, she senses the intrinsic connection to her own Inner Self and recognizes it as an ally in her desire to act as an instrument of healing. Impelled by the intentionality of the healer, the aroused spiritual tension now becomes the leading edge of her personal inner work.

The Experience of the Inner Self

The Inner Self is essentially the soul—the spiritual or innermost part of an individual's being. It is the yearning for self-realization, and it is the impetus of this yearning that carries the therapist to another level of consciousness where awareness of the Inner Self acquires a reality of its own. It is in the process of consciously integrating her Inner Self into the daily routines of her life that the therapist becomes aware that there is not just one reality; there are multiple realities depending upon the aspect of consciousness on which she chooses to focus. It is in integrating these multiple realities that the illumination may click! on: I believe that it is the Inner Self that is evolving and that the TT therapist often becomes aware of this transformation. The persona is merely the container for the experiences that evoke that evolution. The healer recognizes that she needs to remain well grounded, deeply centered, consciously mindful of the inferences of her actions, and accepting of that responsibility as she allows her inner life to permeate the persona of her outer life. In so doing, the practice of Therapeutic Touch now becomes a transpersonal act, and healing becomes a committed life way.

There are certain indicators of the Inner Self that have endured through time, which are experienced by the TT therapist. Early in her practice she becomes aware of a substantial increase in accessible personal knowledge, an interior knowing that can be trusted. This awareness is introduced by a felt shift in consciousness that serves to introduce a sensibility to nonphysical cues. Several things seem to happen at once; there is a calming and quieting of her physical body and a unique stillness seems to permeate the surrounding atmosphere. She feels a sense of peace, of equilibrium and well-being.

There is also a sense of timelessness, as if time is no longer an appropriate consideration. The healer's perception deepens; she may experience the nonlinear as waves, spirals, mobius happenings, and other impressions often difficult to put into words. Synchronicity enters her life and power appears, but on its own terms. There is an irrepressible welling up of desire to elevate her behavior, to surmount disabilities and negative patterns of demeanor, to overcome crises, and to realize a sense of direction to her life. Thus the gifts of the Inner Self resemble those stimulated by the serious practice of sustained centering, but extend past the enactment of the TT process into daily life happenings.

As the quest for self-realization deepens and the therapist's practice of Therapeutic Touch continues and becomes full-fledged, she finds that her frequent TT practice invites a psychological and spiritual transformation.

Making Friends with the Inner Self

Issie is a metaphor and moniker for one's Inner Self (IS),* for who we really are as individual beings. For example, Issie is:

- *The blueprint for my survival,*
- *The idea of my self-preservation,*

---

*Some years ago, as part of a presentation at one of the mentorship programs at Camp Indralaya, Orcas Island, Washington, students began referring to the Inner Self—a term that had been adopted by Dora Kunz—as IS, which evolved into the humorous and affectionate term "Issie." Dr. Krieger became fond of this nickname, and she composed this poem. —*Editor*

- *The roots of my self-esteem,*
- *The limits of my interests.*

Within the concept of Issie lies the power of self. For instance, Issie is:

- *The dynamism of my energy's deep source.*
- *It encompasses the faculty of my foresight, my potential wisdom.*
- *From it springs the potency for my ability to help, to heal.*

Issie is:

- *My ally, my friend,*
- *My guide,*
- *My teacher,*
- *My most inner self.*

Issie IS.

Experientially Acknowledging the Friendly Inner Self

A sustained state of centered consciousness, unusual in our hurry-up time, is the focal point around which the practice of Therapeutic Touch revolves and the grounded source from which it gains its power. Through experience we come to realize that Therapeutic Touch is an opportunity to touch another level of consciousness, a new path of self-realization of our ability to compassionately help those in need. We enter an inner journey toward what we are in the depth of our being. As has been stated, this understanding comes with the conscious liaison with the healer's Inner Self. If the healer is doing Therapeutic Touch correctly, she will not be personally attached to the outcome of the interaction, for she is calling upon a source other than her self-willed persona.

The consistent practice of sustained centering sensitizes the therapist to a recognition of the subtle world of the nonphysical. Very frequently the TT therapist, in an effort to understand this new perspective, will intensify her inner work in ways such as adopting the practice of meditation. Self-search practices reinforce her growing relationship with her most enduring self. As this affinity ripens, Inner Self becomes a trusted ally, friend, teacher, and reliable guide, and the therapist's healing practice becomes more focused and coherent. This indicates a significant shift in perception that sensitizes her to higher orders of self, which now begin to act in her daily life.

What the healer is trying to do is reach beyond the usual locked-in viewpoint of things-as-they-are, and attempt to align with the more unrestrained perspective of her Inner Self. Now it becomes a different kind of intelligence one pursues, a perception beyond the six basic physical senses; it becomes a transpersonal healing as she becomes more acutely aware of the deep inner work to which she now has access, fulfilled and potentiated by her own Inner Self. In this deep-seated stretch to actualize personal potential for insightful and creative healing in the service of those in need, she perceives for herself the opportunity for significant transformative change, as that change is reflected in the quality of her healing interactions and also in her own life events.

This state often becomes noticeable to the TT therapist as she initially finds herself consciously aware of the need to help someone who is ill or injured, and then intentionally engages her sense of compassion-in-action to offer a healing session with that person. The therapist often begins to realize that change in her life events seem to be accelerating. Less obvious to the therapist herself—although it may be noticeable to others—is that she, too, has been going through a fine-tuned but transforming change.

Sometimes it is possible to catch a glimpse of the Inner Self by becoming aware of one's own mood. In our culture we often think of mood as a descriptor of our attitude, disposition, or temperament; however, mood is also a deep feeling, a state of mind dominated by a particular emotion. Feelings may be experienced as amorphous, undeveloped, and ill-defined. However, with diligence it is possible to tease back sensations and capture some sense of its content. Most frequently this information will settle back into the unconscious, but with perseverance and sensitivity it can be coaxed to conscious awareness. It is then that the healer can begin to realize the extent of the reach of her own mindset, whose perspective is now so closely aligned with her Inner Self.

Intuition offers insight into linkage with the Inner Self. Intuition has been a singular, incisive factor in my own life. In trying to understand its processes, my observation is that like a muscle that one exercises, the potency of intuition increases with use, and although intuition thrives on uncontrived spontaneity, its accuracy sharpens under the lens of objective analysis. To test it, I simply follow its prompts every time (except twice in my lifetime, for which I later kicked myself very hard). This can be difficult if our intuitive action is against a majority view, therefore a good understanding or informed acceptance of our underlying convictions is important.

Serendipity and synchronicity may both enter one's life smoothly and unobtrusively as the Inner Self actively engages the person's life way. Serendipity is often defined as an accidental discovery, or a stumbling upon exactly the right thing at the right moment; synchronicity applies to significant events, simultaneous and seemingly related but without a cause-and-effect relationship, happening in close conjunction or occurring at the same time. I have no rationale for these happenings, and that may be the answer: they are not rational. I can live with that. I accept that there are multiple realities, and it is nice to envision that the universe is behind my efforts, even if unbeknownst to me.

Since the evidence of a subtle reflection of the healer's Inner Self becomes clarified through a committed, sustained centering of consciousness—and such a proposition is supported by events occurring in the everyday happenings of her daily life—I urge that such occurrences be encouraged to go one step further. We recognize that the healee also has an Inner Self. During the healing session the therapist is encouraged to act as though this is an accepted reality. In other words, the suggestion is that during the healing interaction, as the healer feels herself deeply centered and in touch with her Inner Self, she brings the energy of intentionality into play and purposefully attempts to communicate mind-to-mind with the Inner Self of the healee. From this more impersonal stance she can reflect and perhaps open up for the healee a glimpse or an impression of his own Inner Self.

How one fully engages this mindful act is difficult to describe, but the basic steps involve at least two factors: the healer needs a reliable sense of that inner connection as this experience plays through her consciousness and, most necessarily, she needs the ability to translate that comprehension into a clear communication, mind-to-mind, with what she perceives to be a similar state of consciousness in the healee. The operative words in these instructions are "a clear communication." The actual process is much like what occurs during mental telepathy; however, intentionality is called upon to make it an acutely conscious experience. During the mind-to-mind communication the healer may offer a direct, nonverbal message to the Inner Self of the client. Ultimately, this mind-to-mind communication depends on the willingness of the healee to engage; we have learned that this silent permission from the field of the healee may come more from his heart, his own experience of sentience, rather than from his conscious mind.

There is no simple way of knowing the client's private agenda concerning his illness; however, silently and gently done, there is nothing about the attempt to contact his Inner Self that will do harm, and therefore it is worth a try. In those instances where the Inner Self of the client is open to the message from the healer, the healing process can be unusually effective and surprisingly rapid. This effect is not magical; rather, it reinforces the notion that all healing is self-healing.

Finally, I will note a most reliable way of detecting Inner Self in your life, and that is by becoming more sensitive to the changes occurring in your worldview, your lifestyle, your aspirations, and your passions. As I noted, others may become aware of these signs of vibrant transformation in you before you do, for this shift in consciousness is frequently so deep-seated and unobtrusive that your own spontaneous utterances may be the first to call this ongoing shift in consciousness to your attention. It is only then that you realize the profound nature of your fine-tuned inner engagement in this transforming process.

A useful exercise to reinforce this awakening is offered below; however, it rests on an ability used in TT practice, "deep listening," which therefore is offered first:

@ Suggestions for Becoming Acutely Aware through Deep Listening

Materials: pen and paper (keep nearby)

Suggested procedure:

1. Begin by taking a few gentle, deep breaths and settling into your seat so that you feel comfortable.

2. For two minutes, close your eyes or use "soft eyes." Go beyond or beneath the disturbance of any outside noises; let them continue, but simply do not pay attention to them.

3. Now, quiet the demands of the incessant chatter of your brain; let it do what it has to do, but do not pay undue attention to it. Let it do its thing—but for two minutes you have more important things needing your attention.

4. Time-travel beyond the chatter by listening very deeply and intently to the stillness within you. Give over to that nonphysical, energetic space at the edge of your sense of time-in-between (which naturally occurs briefly outdoors at twilight and daybreak), and let this perfect stillness wash over you. Just concentrate on deeply listening; it can become an *open sesame* for your personal time-in-between.

5. As an idea or a phrase comes to mind, without opening your eyes or disturbing your mood, reach over to the nearby pen and paper and jot down your thought.

6. Continue deep listening. Linger in this inner quietude that is not time-bound. It is a place neither of space as we know it nor of time in its usual guises; nevertheless, maintain a silent but discerning alertness for its subtle messages.

7. Accept this novel shift in consciousness and enjoy the many new avenues of thought and genial encounters of a different kind that it offers. Say *yes!* to the universe and its other-worldly perspective.

8. When you are ready, move an arm or a foot and come back to everyday waking consciousness at a comfortable pace.

9. Write down any significant thoughts, expressions, symbols, ideas, and so on.

10. Label this exercise "An Out-of-Body Experience!" and put its realizations into action in your life happenings.

@ Sleeping with the Inner Self

Materials needed:

- Reading materials on the Inner Self and on deep listening*
- Blank sheets of paper and a pen (keep nearby)

Suggested procedure:

1. Before falling asleep, read material on the Inner Self and on deep listening.
2. As you prepare yourself for sleep, turn your attention to your breathing. Don't change the way you are breathing, just notice that you are breathing; that is, be relaxed and yet alert to the natural rhythm of your breathing.
3. If your attention floats away, gently bring the focus of your mind back to the rhythm of your breathing again and again as necessary. The rhythm of your breathing will reassert itself quickly and easily; all you need to do is turn your attention to an effortless deep listening of the quiet rhythm of your breathing.
4. Go with the rhythm and softly say to yourself *breathing in* with each inhalation, and *breathing out* with each exhalation. At the same time, clearly visualize your Inner Self as a streaming of clear light that illumines from within the shifting of the rhythmic waves of your breathing.
5. Drifting with these words and this visualization of clear light, permit yourself to slip into sleep.
6. In the morning simply note your mood upon awakening. Continue to lie quietly and expand your sense of the feeling of that mood.
7. Quietly observe how it feels to be wafted slowly to full consciousness. Bring back with you images, emotions, symbols, memories, a word or a phrase, a special language, or a few notes of music that you can hum to yourself.
8. As you fully awaken, write down whatever you remember.

---

*For materials on the Inner Self, see Dolores Krieger, *Therapeutic Touch as Transpersonal Healing* (Seattle, Wash.: SeaChange Health and Wellness, 2017), 114–27; Krieger, *Therapeutic Touch Inner Workbook* (Rochester, Vt.: Bear & Company, 1996), 138–42; Dora Kunz with Dolores Krieger, *The Spiritual Dimension of Therapeutic Touch* (Rochester, Vt.: Bear & Company, 2004), 199–200. For deep listening, see *Therapeutic Touch Inner Workbook*, 148 ("Listening to the Deep Dee"), or any spiritual teachings that are meaningful to you. —*Editor*

Note: By deeply listening and striving to be sensitive to your Inner Self you also are opening to the opportunity to change the neural circuitry of your brain, the gateway to your consciousness. You will know it is happening by your increased sensitivity to and effortless stretching of your own boundaries of awareness and of those in need of healing.

The very act of believing that the inner life is accessible lends courage and decisive purpose to life activities. Life may become more demanding and even confrontational, but with Inner Self as ally and acknowledged mentor of each individual TT therapist's experiment in self-exploration, life becomes highly and personally meaningful, and deeply satisfying. Be compassionate to those in need. Be gentle with yourself. Living the healing way is a very long trail. Ho!

5

Giving Voice to Assumptions

Assumptions, by definition, are beliefs and expectations that we take for granted. Their presence is often so subtle that we don't realize they lend us an overview of the particular reality upon which we base our ideas about healing as process, how it works, and what can be accomplished with it.

Major Assumptions underlying the TT Process

It is true that the way of the healer has most often been drawn from oral teachings traditionally handed down through the centuries, teacher to student; or in the mysterious way of personal introspection, the knowing way of the healer has been drawn out of one's own psychic depths. Either way, the deep background of hunches, inferences, or assumptions we have had reaches back to healings of ancient times, which hold the secrets of the validity of healing. It is to these assumptions that we now turn our full attention.

When we bring our awareness to the underlying assumptions we are able to view the operational groundwork from which the healing process arises. Therefore, identifying the major assumptions will simultaneously acknowledge the limits, biases, or reservations we may have about the theoretical frame we will ultimately construct. At some later date,

51

should someone pick up on the hypotheses, question them, and then put into effect a test of these hypotheses under controlled conditions—and if that research confirms these suppositions—we can then move toward the validation of the healing practice and the clarification of these ideas and concepts that we use to explain what happens during a session. First comes a recognition of those assumptions.

Major assumptions that underlie the healing process are intrinsically bound to the reality of the therapist; as noted, they are the lens through which she regards her healing work, its limitations, its opportunities, and its essential meaning. There are additional assumptions that have accrued at the foundations of the healing way—inferences, surmises, and presumptions that may have shed a bit of light at a critical moment. Of these many, at this time we will choose for scrutiny only four of the central assumptions about the healing process:

1. Healing is a natural human potential that can be actualized under appropriate circumstances.
2. Essentially, the enactment of the healing process within the therapist is transpersonal.
3. In grave illnesses and trauma a person's destiny may delimit the possible effects of treatment with healing.
4. There are intangible networks of intelligent and dynamic forces that underlie natural human functions as they relate to the healing process.

Major Assumption #1

Healing is a natural human potential that can be actualized under appropriate circumstances.

Early in the practice of Therapeutic Touch a distinction was realized between the terms "healing" and "curing," which are frequently thought of as synonyms, although the words themselves have different derivations. The term "cure" comes from the Latin word *cura,* meaning to remedy or to get rid of an ailment or evil. It refers to a course of medical treatment, a panacea. The word "heal," however, comes from the Anglo-Saxon word *haelen*—to make whole—and is further defined as "to make healthy, to bring into harmony."

Healing has to do with how we think of ourselves, our worldview or philosophy of life; it implies an enhancement of the quality of life. Fundamentally, to cure is to care for, but to heal means to care about, which implies liking or affection.*

In the English language there are many connotations of the term "healing," which can clarify several of the dimensions of that term, as are listed below:

CONNOTATIONS OF THE WORD "HEAL"

Connotation	Definition
Alleviate	To lessen or make less severe
Attune	To adjust (a person or a thing) to a situation
Harmonize	To make or form a consistent whole
Integrate	To combine diverse elements into a whole
Invigorate	To give strength to
Mend	To restore to a sound condition
Nourish	To enrich, to promote the development of
Rebuild	To build again or differently
Recuperate	To recover from illness, exhaustion, loss, trauma
Regenerate	To bring into renewed existence
Relieve	To bring or provide aid or assistance to
Revivify	To restore to animation, activity, or life

Fundamentals Used during the Healing Practice
A minimal listing of basic variables that the TT therapist uses during the practice of healing includes:

- Compassion as power
- Sustained centering

---

*Dolores Krieger, *Therapeutic Touch as Transpersonal Healing* (Seattle, Wash.: SeaChange Health and Wellness, 2017), 196.

- Some aspect of laying on of hands
- Therapeutic use of the vital-energy and psychodynamic fields of both the healer and the healee
- Work at the transpersonal level between the Inner Self of healer and healee
- Techniques of deep visualization
- Mind-to-mind communion between the healer and healee
- Knowledgeable use of the therapist's own chakra complex

The Relationship between the Healer and the Universal Healing Field

As Dora Kunz always reminded our students: "The outcome is not in our hands." This reminder is intrinsic to the intention held by the healer, as she continues to express a deeply compassionate regard for the recipient's well-being. Balanced in this way, the TT therapist is able to act as an instrument of the healing energy and stay detached from the results of the session.

The universal healing field's chief characteristics are based in principles of order, intelligence, and compassion. From my own experience I believe that the press of pranic streaming that surges purposefully from the universal field to and through the TT therapist is imprinted in her body language, gestures, and moods; these features can be perceived objectively by an observer and by the therapist herself. There are several indicators of this state of consciousness, most apparently:

- Receptivity and responsiveness to others' subtle energies, particularly those who are in need. It is this flexibility and ease of mobility in her vital-energy field that allows the therapist to resonate so reliably with the client's needs, and with continued experience it also fosters her ability to be present to her own deeper states of consciousness.
- An ability to have an inner confidence in the client's potentialities in reference to his wholeness and his ability to act in an integrated fashion.
- The ability to focus with a confidence firmly built on her knowl-

edgeable intentionality in directing and modulating the streaming of several subsystems of prana to meet the needs of the client.

- The expression of compassion as a natural corollary to her worldview, and the willingness to be sensitive to the ways compassion for others affects her own lifestyle.
- A conscious recognition of her relationship with the universal healing field. This is most often seen in the therapist's growing awareness of the principles of order that underlie the healing process.

These abilities are integral to the TT therapist's function as a healer—abilities that lie within each person whose potential becomes actualized with training and practice. It is important that the healer "exercises" her vital-energy field to keep it pliable, supple, and accessible. Several such exercises suggest themselves:

- Permitting herself spontaneous acts of compassion, love, sympathy, empathy, and kindness
- Considered (mindful) projections to others of thoughts of peace, calmness, and gentleness
- Meditation, particularly in reference to clear visualizations that seek to increase sensitivity to others in need

Clinical Considerations of the Healing Process

When we studied how the TT process plays itself out between the subtle-energy systems of the healer and the healee, it became clear that there are at least two other less obvious but significant factors involved: one, what emotions the therapist (consciously or unconsciously) might be projecting to the healee, such as anxiety, apprehension, uncertainty; and two—most important—how the healee accepts the therapist's assistance. However, under the best of conditions the healee assimilates the healing energies, which rapidly (on the average, within four minutes) serve to evoke a relaxation response, reduce pain, and rebalance the flow of vital and psychodynamic energies.

Additionally, these healing energies could help disperse sites of energetic congestion, which plays a large part in arousing pain, or diffuse emotional blockages that interfere with the healing processes, particularly of psychosomatic illnesses. We further realized that healing is individual for each person and that there are multiple permutations of the energy that may be sent by the healer; conversely, the field of the healee will assimilate what resonates for him in that moment. Over time we deepened our understanding and appreciation that illness could be about destiny, as well as unhealthy habit patterns and certain genetic propensities in the healee's history. (This is addressed in Major Assumption #3.)

As the practice of Therapeutic Touch becomes a significantly frequent marker of the healer's lifestyle, she begins to exercise the deeper dimensions of her Inner Self. This heightened, therapeutic use of self potentiates previously latent abilities within the therapist, which then may actualize. As these new behaviors are repeated, over time they make a powerful impression on the flows of her subtle-energy fields, and the fields themselves begin to repattern. It is in this manner that committed Therapeutic Touch practice may often facilitate transformation for the TT therapist.

Actualizing Natural Human Potential through the Therapeutic Touch Process

There appears to be a natural progression to these changes within the TT therapist. I will review the phases of the TT process with the focus on what is happening within the therapist. It should be noted that this perspective can be used as a template to evaluate the process of potential becoming actualized. The therapist's personal experience of the phases will vary according to the length of time each one has been practicing. The account of an individual who went through training a few months ago will contrast with the depth of the account by a TT therapist who has been consistently practicing for months or years. This can be observed in the case studies in the study "Looking Over My Shoulder" in part 2.

First Phase: A Call of Compassion and Centering

The therapist is moved initially by a call of compassion to help or heal someone in need. This compassionate intention galvanizes the powers of the therapist's heart chakra at the subtle-energy level, and soon thereafter at the physical level. From my observations the body systems that become involved are the central nervous, cardiovascular, and deep limbic. The first substantive action in which the TT therapist engages is an act of sustained centering of her consciousness.

Second Phase: Approach and Outreach
As has been explained, the therapist continues in the centered state. Since TT is a multitask act, it is during this time as she is starting to interact with the healee that the therapist is also involved in a self-exploration of her own consciousness. This exploration serves to awaken her to the reality of her own Inner Self, who may act as a guide during the healing interaction.

Third Phase: Search/Assessment
Staying on center, using her hand chakras as probes, the therapist engages in a shift in consciousness, a search of the healee's subtle-energy fields to determine the nature of any imbalances and dysrhythmias and how she might help him. In this evaluation, although she may physically touch (with the permission of the healee), most often the search is done by directing with mindful intentionality her nonphysical hand chakras to pass through the healee's subtle-energy fields, just a few inches from the surface of his body. As the therapist progresses in her development, her intuition will become more and more active in the search phase.

The therapist can now easily pick up cues of imbalance in the subtle-energy flows as irregular patterns that are embedded in the healee's vital-energy field. She may perceive cues in his psychodynamic field as well. In some instances the input of multiple cues may offer a vivid visualization of the cause of these imbalances, possibly suggesting how the illness developed. Thus, the practice of the search can become an act of lucid sensitivity training. The clear visualizations that are possible during this phase indicate that primarily her brow chakra is being called upon to function.

Fourth Phase: Rebalance and Reassessment
On the basis of information gathered during the search phase, the therapist decides how to help the ill person rebalance his subtle-energy

fields. In the act of rebalancing the therapist uses her ability to focus with resolute intentionality on the healing effect she wishes to project by the sensitive modulation of the field of the patient; this assistance has been described as "unruffling" and "clearing and balancing." The other technique used in rebalancing is the direction of energy. The therapist is aware that she is connected to the universal healing field and she may decide to offer this energy to the patient. She does this by inviting these subtle energies from the universal field to move through her field, to and through the field of the ill person.

This is done in a mind-to-mind fashion from the therapist to the healing partner. It is possible that the therapist involves the further use of her brow chakra, and that the intuitive guidance from her Inner Self seems to involve her crown chakra.

Fifth Phase: Done/Complete

As the therapist matures in her development, the nature of this phase changes significantly. In the early days of her practice she most likely follows a linear sequence as she has been taught; for example, the done phase may be the second time she touches the feet of the healee or some other conscious thought that guides her. Over time she will come to trust her intuition, the voice of her Inner Self, as she moves from a linear approach to one that is more simultaneous, in which she begins to follow her own inner prompts, guided by the changes she perceives in the fields in each unique TT interaction.

It is the accumulated effect of the therapist's frequent practice of Therapeutic Touch that sculpts the pranic flows in her vital-energy and psychodynamic fields and often transforms her in the process. And we suggest that this experience of transformation is shared by those practicing other healing modalities. On the basis of experience, it seems that the more deeply the therapist can delve into the healing process, the more effective can be her ability to help or to heal those in need. Importantly, there is a deepening connection of the therapist's Inner Self as her healing practice becomes a more consistent part of her life way.

Intermixed with this reorientation, curious questions begin to present themselves to the therapist, focused around the query: What have we allowed to happen to ourselves as this luminous shining—our Inner Self—has patterned and repatterned the pranic streaming, the vital source of our consciousness? Often other questions follow rapidly as the therapist becomes more engaged in the healing act.

What Have We Allowed to Happen?

In an effort to understand the inner process of the healer it helps to consider specific questions that may assist in replicating the experience:

- What have we been dealing with that has the power to initiate such transformation?
- What were the crucial variables involved in the healing moment that allowed this to happen?
- What "just happened"? Could we truly call it a conscious process?
- What "really" (physically or evidentially) happened during those many healing moments?
- What does it actually feel like to be guided by Inner Self?
- Do we do TT, or does TT "do" us?

Moving into the Realm of Transformation

Over time, as we continued to study the responses of our students to the effects of the practice, teaching, and research of Therapeutic Touch, we became more discerning of the dynamics of the process in action. Of prime importance was the growing realization that the verbal expression of healing strongly depended on experiential knowledge based on sentience—the power of perception by the senses rather than structured logic—to articulate clearly this world of interiority, a profound, far-reaching realm into which the student is plunged as she follows a personal commitment to support those who aroused her compassion. Here in the throes of that commitment, in the midst of the healing act itself, the healer is strongly guided by her Inner Self. The language of this profound experience is richly multitasked and multitiered, sentient and proprioceptive, intuitive and instinctive, intentional and willful, and subject to uncommon and unusual hints and hunches about the possible.

As we began to see, at about this stage of one's development in the discipline of Therapeutic Touch the process itself begins to slip away from ordinary reality. It is also about this time that we began to realize that healer and healee are having two very different experiences. From her perspective, the mindful TT therapist may decide to seek out communion Inner Self to Inner Self with the client. The healing enactment now has the opportunity to play itself out at the transpersonal level. It is this intense experiential knowing that guides the committed therapist in her aspiration to heal.

The "Within" Experience of the Healer

The enactment of the healing interaction is clothed in an array of scenarios that facilitate the patterning and repatterning of the pranic flow, keenly overseen by the therapist's Inner Self. When I think of Inner Self, I keep in mind that through time she has represented attributes of the feminine principle that are present in both genders, and that she has always been associated with the flows of life-energy and healing.

There is a natural streaming from the Inner Self of the within toward the ego-focused self who deals with the outer physical world. For these two parts of Self to truly understand each other they need the common language of sentience. Achieving fluency with this language enables the therapist to develop new powers of receptivity and to encourage impressions from her intuition. Simultaneously in the within there is a felt movement, a decided transition of consciousness particularly in her heart and *ajna* (third eye, or brow) chakras as the therapist becomes more self-aware. Access to the mind deepens and becomes more direct, intuition sharpens, and one's ability to concentrate shifts to a more intense level of focus. Behavior changes, perceptions more fully adjust to the within, the therapist feels an irrepressible desire to enter inner spheres of inquiry, and there is an arousal and activation of self-awakening toward a new modeling of the therapist in this realm.

This transformation is made possible by the increasingly close communion that occurs between the therapist and her Inner Self as she intently and compassionately practices, practices, practices Therapeutic Touch for those in need. This empowering assistance is particularly noticeable during the state of sustained centering.

It is because of the committed, vital assistance permitted by this intimate association that the act of sustained centering is considered a true mark of the authenticity of the healing process. It is during this time that the therapist's consciousness is in a state of balance and equipoise, and at one with her Inner Self. She is in the impersonal space where she may become a clear instrument for the universal healing field and remain detached from the outcome. This finely tuned state creates a singular atmosphere that allows the Inner Self to commune with the therapist and enter her daily activities.

This transmission between the TT therapist and her Inner Self has its own language born of sentience, the nature of which has been caught so sensitively by Karen Jaenke: "Something within the soul is stirred when soul language is spoken. . . . The language of the soul reverberates and touches a profound longing within the soul to be addressed in its native tongue."*

Major Assumption #2

Essentially, the enactment of the Therapeutic Touch healing process from the "within" of the Therapeutic Touch therapist is transpersonal.

The transpersonal perspective was an outgrowth of the humanistic psychology movement that Abraham Maslow, psychologist and founder of humanistic psychology, perceived as "the third force." The other two acknowledged psychological forces at that time were psychoanalysis and behaviorism; the third force evolved in response to what some psychologists felt were limitations of both behaviorism and Freudian theory. Transpersonal psychology followed as the fourth force, and its focus was on the inner realms of being, the "within" of de Chardin. One of its avenues of interest was in reference to intuitive explanations of human

---

*Karen Jaenke, "Soul and Soullessness," *ReVision* (Winter 2010): 9.

consciousness; these are based on quite different assumptions from those of the "hard" sciences, particularly in reference to the fundamental nature of the universe. In fact, transpersonal conceptions were the first to significantly break through the established mechanistic frame of reference to which science had been bonded.

The notions of the transpersonal were popularized by Abraham Maslow and Anthony Sutich,* and included within their purview individual spiritual, global, and universal concerns. Jeanne Achterberg, a leading research psychologist and popular author, coined the term "Transpersonal Medicine" as a new system of medicine.

The term "transpersonal"—beyond the persona—refers to events beyond the limits of the as-usual perception of everyday reality. It provides a perspective for the nonordinary and signifies that there are multiple realities.† Jeanne Achterberg wrote, "The common element in most transpersonal healing is that both patient and healer enter into a state of consciousness that is unlike the usual, wide-awake state associated with active thought. The state is often referred to as a trance, an altered or nonordinary state of consciousness, a meditative mind, or some special brainwave frequency, such as is associated with alpha or theta brainwaves."‡

In keeping with this perspective the nursing theorist Jean Watson developed her Theory of Transpersonal Caring. In her words: "The terms transpersonal and a transpersonal caring relationship are foundational to the work. Transpersonal conveys a concern for the inner-life world and subjective meaning of another who is fully embodied. But transpersonal also energetically goes beyond the ego-self and beyond the given moment, reaching to the deeper connections to spirit and with the broader universe. Thus, a transpersonal caring relationship moves beyond ego-self and radiates to spiritual, even cosmic, concerns and connections that tap into healing possibilities and potentials.

---

*A quadriplegic from childhood, Anthony Sutich was a lesser known but equally important figure in both the humanistic and transpersonal psychology movements of the 1960s and '70s. —Editor

†Dolores Krieger, *Therapeutic Touch as Transpersonal Healing* (Seattle, Wash.: SeaChange Health and Wellness, 2017), 15.

‡Krieger, *Therapeutic Touch as Transpersonal Healing,* xv.

"Transpersonal caring seeks to connect with and embrace the spirit or soul of the other through the processes of caring and healing and being in authentic relation, in the moment. Such a transpersonal relationship is influenced by the caring consciousness and intentionality, and energetic presence of the nurse as she enters into the life space or phenomenal field of another person and is able to detect the other person's condition of being (at the soul or spirit level). It implies a focus on the uniqueness of self and other, and the uniqueness of the moment wherein the coming together is mutual and reciprocal, each fully embodied in the moment, while paradoxically capable of transcending the moment, open to new possibilities. The transpersonal nurse has the ability to center consciousness and intentionality on caring, healing, and wholeness, rather than on disease, illness, and pathology."*

Although healing has been a valued human function for tens of thousands of years, the healer consistently has had difficulty in translating the transpersonal experience she has undergone during the healing act into a meaningful communion with someone who is naïve about the healing experience. The major reason for this is that Western culture has adhered to rules of analysis that have depended on Aristotelian if-then logic and laws of probability, although healing practices themselves are realized and personally verified on the basis of experiential knowing, sentience, or mindfulness during the practice of transpersonal healing. It is experiential knowing that informs the therapist of the healee's moment-to-moment states of mind. In this healing act, personal knowledge flows out of sentient acts of compassion, communications from the senses that are discerning, insightful, and often penetratingly clear.

I have applied the term "transpersonal healing" in describing Therapeutic Touch because from my perspective, it is the therapist's Inner Self that empowers the healing process, as compassion as power is expressed during the interaction. This opens the door for the therapist to achieve an intimate relationship with her Inner Self, which acts

---

*Jean Watson and Terri Kaye Woodward, *Jean Watson's Theory of Human Caring: Nursing Theories and Nursing Practice,* 3rd ed., Marilyn E. Parker, Marlaine C. Smith, eds. (Philadelphia: F. A. Davis Co., 2010), 356–57.

as her ally, teacher, and guide during the healing session. It is through this close relationship that the Inner Self "oversees" the therapist's inner work. Since its development as a healing approach, Therapeutic Touch has been shown to be direct, simple, and straightforward—possible to be learned and practiced by anyone, as affirmed by the first major assumption, that healing is a natural human potential. In addition, over time we have come to understand that the process can call out significant nonordinary shifts in consciousness in the therapist to the extent that although the techniques are seemingly simple, the committed use of TT is neither simplistic nor obvious.

In understanding TT as a transpersonal healing modality, we most effectively get a sense of it by defining the idea, giving it a name, symbolizing or otherwise representing it, mapping it, and stating its distinctions. TT can be viewed as a multiplicity of separate things—the phases of call, approach, outreach, search, rebalance, done. However, the healee experiences the underlying wholeness of these combined streams of consciousness both during the formal session and often after the session has ended. The logical exploration of the parts that make up the whole of TT is necessary, but we take care to avoid a reductionist approach, ever mindful of the essential characteristic of the process—an interaction with the life-sustaining pranic flow, the vital-energy streaming that, in some still-unknown manner, responds to human consciousness and supports healing in sentient beings.

It is my personal impression that at the core of Therapeutic Touch lies the challenge of confronting one's own being. I find such opportunities for deep self-inquiry stimulating, even exhilarating. My guess is that it gives me an invaluable means for alignment with my Inner Self. Essentially, as I have previously noted, this is done by setting up favorable circumstances to work consciously with her. TT practice offers a rich opportunity for such singular engagement. Consistent, compassionate, and committed practice of Therapeutic Touch attracts one's better angels, giving the transpersonal an opportunity to emerge. Through personal experimentation with the transpersonal, the willingness for self-exploration can lead us to know, truly know, for ourselves. We realize in a very personal way that within the context of Therapeutic

Touch, healing is a conscious, full engagement of the Inner Self in the compassionate interest of being fully present to someone who is ill, in trauma, or in energy deficit. Additionally, this personal realization may be experienced by healers of other disciplines.

It has been the experience with many TT therapists that engagement with the healing process may effect change in some of the following: one's worldview, lifestyle, life goals, and how one conducts one's life. Indeed, this shift in consciousness may significantly affect priorities, motivations, and drives.

In sum, Therapeutic Touch offers transformation. A major reason that modes of energy healing unfold so easily into the transpersonal realm is because healing is primarily experiential. Its focus and direction arise within the therapist as she becomes aware of, and consciously seeks out, her Inner Self. As noted, Therapeutic Touch by its very nature offers personal transformation, and as a natural consequence the healer now lives in a world of multiple realities and countless opportunities to plunge her own psychological and spiritual depths of being.

We know that TT can interface with all therapeutic modalities and medical procedures. In the world of energy healing there are disciplines—such as massage, chiropractic, acupuncture, and acupressure—that include physical contact to a greater degree than Therapeutic Touch, which relies on the nonphysical chakras and the altered state of consciousness of sustained centering.

It is the consistent practice of Therapeutic Touch and its crucial need to be performed against a background of sustained centering of the therapist's consciousness that invites the involvement of her higher chakras, her more finely structured, coherent centers of consciousness. This centered state of consciousness allows the therapist to extend her awareness into the farther reaches of the network of pranic flows that vitalize the human body. According to the ancient literature of many cultures, these pranic flows are actually a stratum of what we in the West call "stream of consciousness." Over the years of practice and teaching of Therapeutic Touch we have observed that the process begins to invite students into a way of awakening within a deep, coherent understanding of certain of these pranic flows. When it is realized that these vitalizing streamings, under the drive of compassion, are able to help someone who is ill, wounded, or in trauma, then the student begins to understand how the healing process is so significantly affected by the functions of the therapist's mind.

As has been noted, an atmosphere is evoked during sustained centering, which initiates the TT practice. It is the continuance of this state of consciousness that provides the inner milieu, the spiritual tension that is attractive to the descent of the healer's Inner Self into her daily activities. For the compassionate healer, awareness of this pranic flow is now quickened, and its functioning is enhanced with her continued practice.

One of the results that can occur in this transpersonal space of the TT session is that the healee begins to understand the process that is helping him. He may know intellectually of the first major assumption, that healing is a natural human potential; or he may intuit this through his lived experience. He may then come to understand that whatever the healer is doing, he can learn to do also, should he wish to do so. Particularly if his condition is improving under treatment, she may become his model or mentor in reference to healing, for he can imagine that one day he might be able to do for others what she is doing for him now. This scenario has been played out numerous times since the early days of TT. We have had patients attend classes and come to our camps for their own healing who then later become students, receiving formal training; some of those have gone on to become teachers.

Major Assumption #3

In grave illness and trauma, a person's destiny may delimit the possible effects of treatment with healing.

Today, to an extent not previously possible in Western cultures, individuals committed to consciously accessing their inner lives are able to take the direction for their lives into their own hands, concentrate their intentions and resolutions into meaningful foci, and make their goals and yearnings act as agents of personal change. Limitations and restrictions are remarkably low in this time; however, they must still be taken into account.

Destiny is a word that is seldom heard in our still strongly mechanistic era. Destiny implies a goal, and the end point of goal-setting assumes decision. Decision presumes judgment, and judgment presupposes meaning. Unfortunately our time—as I write—is chaotic; our society of the majority is wildly searching for meaning. In contradistinction to the more holistic thrust of this Newer Age, traditional Western civilization posits that we live in a probabilistic universe of direct cause and effect of physical events. Within that if-then context, it would seem that all events have *raison d'être*. However, the fate of each of us at some time in our lives seems inexplicable. Prediction of foreseeable trends—a faithful standby for the past several centuries for scrying the future—does not always work. Thus when the unexpected enters our lives with an unsettling call for life skills for which we seem totally unprepared, then *Why me?* is the common cry, and the answer may take a lifetime in coming or it simply may evade our understanding, sometimes with consequences for our future health and healing.

Twin notions—the idea of reincarnation and the concept of karma—offer a timeless perspective in which to work through the problems implicit in evolving toward full human potential, which is perhaps why they have been constants in some of the great religions of the world. Although thought by many to be uniquely distinctive of Eastern thought, in the West these teachings were important to Plato and the subsequent Neoplatonic tradition, as well as to the Essenes, some early Christian Gnostic sects, the Kabbalists, and the Hasidim, who carried these ancient ideas and precepts into modern times. Now much that was once esoteric has become an important part of a generalized uprising of spiritual consciousness during the last quarter of the twentieth century, as it continued to meld with the current "Newer" Age of our time.

These beliefs are included as a theoretical explanation for the mysteries of the healing process; they are in no way necessary to accept for the study and practice of Therapeutic Touch.

In addition to our hypothesis of karma as an influence, there are several factors that can restrict healing from taking place or from lasting:

- Destiny, as is noted here in the third major assumption, seems prime.
- There may be a lack of willingness (often not conscious) on the part of the healee to engage himself in the healing process and let it happen.
- The healee may demonstrate an inability to relax or permit others to help him relax so that the healing process can most easily and smoothly permeate his body and energy field.

One of the understandings carried by each TT therapist is that although she may be skilled in her practice, it is always the choice of the healee to experience the relaxation response and to receive the rebalancing. It may be that an expectation—conscious or unconscious—can interfere with the receptive state. This typically does not happen with infants and children who have not formed an expectation.

Many TT therapists have had the experience of reaching out to a patient and then sensing some degree of an energetic boundary surrounding him. That is, the therapist perceives areas in the healing partner's vital-energy field that seem to be enclosed by subtle but real barriers to her intention to assist with rebalancing. Sometimes it is only in the recall phase that the therapist will realize the aspect of an energetic boundary.

Because of the typically high reliability of the healing of psychosomatic problems, the resistance by the field of the patient to the healing energies is significant. It is, of course, always the prerogative of the healee to receive the intervention offered by the therapist or not. But this dynamic can cause us to wonder: could the inability to receive healing be based in something to which we usually do not pay much attention, a subtle factor that falls outside the realm of current scientific credibility, such as the patient's destiny?

Of several possible factors, destiny or the karma of an individual seems the most bewildering, for karmic consequences may act suddenly and simultaneously on several factors in one's life. The major focus of belief in the concept of karma centers on relationships; however, karmic consequences are concerned with three aspects of the individual being:

- It is recognized that one could not bear at one time all the karma of one's past incarnations and so only a part of one's karma is selected for the person to deal with in his present life.
- There remains the rest of the karmic load that will have to be dealt with in the future.
- Finally, there is the karma made anew as present circumstances work through the current time. This also must be dealt with in the future.

Dora Kunz, a lifelong member of the Theosophical Society, spoke to us on the subject of karma from time to time. An independent thinker, Dora would never insist on anyone agreeing with her beliefs:

It is within the patterns that we weave in our lifetimes that we create the ground or basis for the working out of karma. Many people hold a limited view of karma. They think that if I hit you, you will hit me back. That is simplistic; the concept of karma is truly more profound and far-reaching. Karma is not made up only of physical reactions; it reaches deeply into all levels of consciousness. Our interactions and activities at the different levels of consciousness become the root sources and energetic ingredients of karmic forces. They direct how the natural laws of karma and rebirth are manifested within and around us by the circumstances of life. Our deeply held feelings, thoughts, and actions have a tremendous effect, usually through our memory of them. They are what karmically bind us, be they positive feelings such as love and friendship or negative ones of anger, hate, or resentment.*

The concepts of destiny and karma have much in common. Destiny is a more recent Judeo-Christian-Muslim version and is usually thought of as being active within the confines of the present life. The belief in karma, however, is considered most usually within the context of several,

---

*Dora Kunz with Dolores Krieger, Ph.D., R.N., *The Spiritual Dimension of Therapeutic Touch* (Rochester, Vt.: Bear & Company, 2004), 67.

even countless lives and, as previously noted, is strongly related to the idea of reincarnation. From our current view, the beliefs of karma and reincarnation are most frequently thought to confer insight on questions such as:

- Who am I?
- Why have I been born into this space and time?
- And in perplexing situations: Why me?

Answers to such queries center around several lines of thought, such as:

- Inherited genetic factors
- Unexpected life events
- Synchronicity—seemingly accidental or coincidental events that occur in the same space and time

The connecting link between the beliefs of karma and reincarnation embodies the notion that reincarnation grants an opportunity over several lifetimes to learn from significant errors of judgment, limitations of thought, or misconceptions that an individual had in the past. In considering these concepts it is important to think of each situation within the context of the person's worldview at the time, particularly in reference to the social mores then in vogue. In hindsight, the story of a supposed destined event often makes sense.

Considerations of Major Assumption #3 in Clinical Practice

During clinical practice, in ways we do not always understand, the therapist is able to differentiate various subtle-energy signals from several sources:

- Pranic flow
- Psychodynamic-field temperature: an energetic perception described metaphorically as heat or coolness (not physical evidence of temperature differences)
- Texture of subtle-energy fields

- Intrinsic rhythm of subtle-energy fields
- Nonverbal communion, intuition, mind-to-mind, and experiential knowing

Similar to the Inner Self of the patient, the individual karma of the therapist, and the karma of the patient, as well as the combined karma their healing interaction evokes, these unknowns may also set boundaries on the effectiveness of the treatment.

In reference to the healer-healee relationship during the sessions, I would suggest treating the idea of destiny or karma as one possible explanation for instances where there is an inability to restore balance to the field of the healee, or when unforeseen, unaccountable problems arise during the time of the TT process. However, because healing is an intimate interaction, I would also take into account my own side of the equation, my own involvement, and would not treat the question lightly.

I might use the Deep Dee techniques to seek out a level of communication with my healee's Inner Self. I would closely and deeply "listen" to my intuition, and I would be willing to realize that I might not be the one to bring healing to this patient. If I didn't come up with satisfactory findings, or if I felt my understanding were incomplete, I would recognize that I did not have the final answer. I would earnestly try to be wise about my personal involvement or attachment to the situation or the person, so that I would be clear of bias when trying to recognize when, or if, an experience may need to happen for the welfare of my healing partner. I would remain mindful of the option of referring the patient to an appropriate colleague.

Paradoxically, although healing can engage therapeutically with a wide range of physical and emotional problems, I have found that there are some psychosomatic conditions with which I have had limited success. I have also found that certain physical dysfunctions, such as some endocrine problems, may not respond well. However, I would never discourage anyone from offering TT when she receives that call. There may be some barriers of various origins, but every single TT session is unique in time and space and it is always worth a try.

Major Assumption #4

There are intangible networks of intelligent and dynamic forces that underlie normal human functions as they relate to the healing process.

> Our normal working consciousness is but one special type of consciousness while all about it, parted from it by the filmiest of screens, there lie potential forms of consciousness entirely different. We may go through life without suspecting their existence, but apply the requisite stimulus and at a touch they are there, in all their completeness.*

As has been stated, during the development and teaching of Therapeutic Touch we began to see that the practice of sustained centering and the interactions within the transpersonal facilitate the entry of the therapist into these realms described above by William James. This is, in fact, the way that some TT therapists experience the universal healing field.

In the story of David's healing (chapter 3) I related how I connected with the intangible networks through the energies of the animals—the dog and the horses—as well as the "natural energies that were in abundance on this responsive land."

Dora Kunz was very fond of trees and felt they had a deep connection with the practice of healing. At gatherings held in nature she would typically direct us to "look at the trees" before she began her talk. These words from Dora are from *The Spiritual Dimension of Therapeutic Touch*:

> I always feel that trees have a certain consciousness of their own and that when we sit among them there is an exchange in consciousness. They have an enormous abundance of vitality that they freely share, which is compatible with our own energy. In a general sense I believe trees like us to be among them as friends. If you quietly say to them, "I appreciate you," or tell them how beautiful they are, their reaction

---

*William James, *The Varieties of Religious Experience* (London: Longmans, Green, & Co., 1902), 378.

to your thoughts will give you some of their enormous energy. In that way there will be a sort of communication between you and the trees. I sometimes think that visualizing a tree is the easiest therapy of all, for the relationship can affect us deeply and the memory of it can be of great help in times of need.*

A meaningful experience with a tree is also described in chapter 7, case 12: "Connection with Oak Tree Assists Deepening Wholeness" (pages 151–56) in which a TT therapist relates how her energetic connection with a tree enhanced a healing session.

The intangible networks come into play with experiments that have been done on praying, or directing one's thoughts to people, to animals, and to other life forms—plants, seeds, and molds. "Something is happening" in the experiments, such as those conducted by Bernard Grad, a biologist at McGill University in Montreal in the 1960s. Grad had the noted Hungarian healer Oskar Estebany (whom Dora Kunz and I were to later observe) hold beakers of ordinary tap water with the intention of infusing the water with healing energy. That water was then applied to plants that had previously been watered with a one percent saline solution, which would retard normal growth. Although the plants watered with only the saline were affected negatively, "The water energized by Estebany did not produce the negative result. I suggest that the intelligence of the universal field was accessed by Estebany in his intention and that the energy of his intention reached the energy fields of the plants."†

There have been many such experiments, but a recent one performed by IKEA with schoolchildren in the United Arab Emirates at GEMS (Global Educational Management System) schools caught my attention. IKEA took two dracaena plants to these schools for thirty days and instructed the children to verbally bully one plant and to compliment and praise the other. At the end of thirty days the complimented plant

---

*Dora Kunz with Dolores Krieger, Ph.D., R.N., *The Spiritual Dimension of Therapeutic Touch* (Rochester, Vt.: Bear & Company, 2004), 50–51.
†Bernard Grad, "Some Biological Effects of Laying-on of Hands: A Review of Experiments with Animals and Plants," *Journal of the American Society for Psychological Research* 59 (1965): 95–127.

was thriving but the bullied plant was drooping.* This was a demonstration of the power of the energy of word, thought, and intention. In my view, the results were facilitated by the involvement of the intelligent forces of the universal field.

Another interpretation of the intelligences of the universal healing field can be found in the concept of Indra's net. The Hindu god Indra was considered the creator of the universe. He caused a net to be constructed—often visualized as a vast spider's web—containing everything that exists and ever has and ever will. At every juncture of the net is a jewel, each representing the essence of an individual's consciousness or a phenomenon. As Thich Nhat Hanh describes it:

> This is a net made of jewels, and in each jewel you see reflected all the other jewels. Looking into the one you see the all. Suppose you build a hall made of mirrors, and then you enter holding a candle. Looking into a mirror you see you and the candle, and when you turn around you see that each mirror reflects you and the candle in the mirror, too. You just need to look into one mirror to see all the reflections of you and the candle. Countless numbers of you and countless candles are reflected in just one mirror.†

This is a model of the universal field—a representation of unition—to which we are all connected and toward which we can reach out for healing of ourselves and others.

Dora Kunz sometimes spoke to her understanding that angels are a part of the intangible networks.

> Healing happens at many different levels, and many different angelic beings are involved in the healing process. They are most prevalent in cases where significant change is involved, such as from birth to life and from life to death, and then they try to help in every way that they can. The way angels help in healing is not a simple thing. As their world is oriented toward a different time frame than ours, they are of the future. When they help a human being during a time

---

*"Bully a Plant; Say No to Bullying," April 30, 2018, YouTube (website).
†From a Dharma Talk: "The Power of Visualization," June 2004.

of crisis they do so in a way that will be most appropriate for the individual's future.

Angels help with the healing interaction, as in Therapeutic Touch, and with the continuing process of healing itself. They help those who wish to help others by assisting in the projection of healing energy to help the ill person attain peace of mind as well as a healing of the physical body. The angels may be able to help people to have peace of mind even when they have pain.*

Some TT therapists report sensing angelic presences. One person relates: "During TT I sometimes invoke the presence of St. Raphael, the archangel of healing. He represents a powerful energy field that allows me to be an instrument for bringing in his healing potential when doing TT. It is helpful to realize I am not bringing him in as an individual but aligning to his vast energy field. When I am connected to this field I feel that I am filled with the intense cobalt blue light that Dora has described."

Centering as an Entry to Communication with the Intangible Networks

Therapeutic Touch in action is difficult to define coherently because so many levels of consciousness seem to be operating at the same time, but perhaps one can begin to get a hint, an inference, from first looking at this act of transpersonal healing as process. The entry point in TT is the act of centering the consciousness; this state of mind is sustained throughout the entirety of the TT session, even while the therapist simultaneously practices the appropriate skills with her patient. This means, of course, that the TT therapist is in an altered state of consciousness throughout the healing session. It becomes evident over time that it is this state that deeply nurtures and supports the empowerment of the therapist. It is from the centered state that the healer reaches out to the universal healing field, inviting the energies to move through her and through the field of the person in need. Below are some descriptions of the experience of this connection from my files of accounts of TT therapists through the years.

---

*Dora Kunz, *Spiritual Aspect of the Healing Arts* (Wheaton, Ill.: Quest Books, 1985), 225.

- As we focus within and seek out the Inner Self who dwells in the deeper places of our being, we become aware of the sheer pulsations of life and extend our consciousness into the downbeat of their flow and beyond.
- Adjusting to the shift in perception we become cognizant of organized presence or intelligence, focus our attention, and "listen."
- A new avenue of communication—a resonant communion—becomes increasingly apparent and we direct attention inward and more deeply. Mindful not to break this gossamer thread of subtle rapport, we continue to tune in intently and with committed sensitivity for a response.
- We sense a deep-rooted response that arises fluidly from within. It is that which we are seeking, and in this rare time-space it acts as a dimly remembered point of reference for our now keen, intensely focused attention.
- With heightened clarity of purpose we further extend the focus of our centered attention, following the leading edge of response toward higher/deeper levels of consciousness. And effortlessly we "connect": click! and we are in another "place," a singular, altered time frame.
- Seamlessly the energy or "feeling" that comes through is sublimated in a simple act of gentle compassion, as it is lightly fashioned to meet the needs of the patient.
- The TT therapist begins to feel this quest for the healing of the other as an effortless sense of oneness, of bonded unition, as well as an upwelling sense of peace and an unbroken stillness. It is as though a precious aspect of one's Inner Self has been touched and, as always, she is there as irrefutable ally to help or to heal other or self.

The hint that the query "How did I get here?" alludes to Major Assumption #4 is that as the therapist compassionately answers the call from another in need, she sensitizes herself to the universal healing field. This state of awakening previously lay slumbering as a potential deep within her being, an ancient limbic nest of neurochemical antennae. To actualize this potential she shifts into an altered state as she shapes her thoughts into a sustained centering of her consciousness. From this centered state she establishes her connection with whatever she believes to be the healing energies of the universal field; for some this is the experience of communion with the intangible networks. She then reaches out to the flow of prana that forms the matrix of the patient's psychodynamic and mental fields—subtle-energy interactions now streaming between therapist and patient. To make sense of these bits of information that converge, the therapist resorts to her ready, natural access to the language of intuition, whose idiom is available to all humans. This expression becomes accessible as an aspect of sentience, a fine, primary state of perception that often gives voice through body language.

Meanwhile, the urge toward self-awakening, which is coupled to this search for communion, is greatly assisted by the constant presence of compassion-as-power, which has motivated the healing act from its initiation in the therapist's response to the call. This potent mix calls forth in the healer latent psychic and mental abilities that she can now add to her storehouse of effective healing tools, instruments that are much used as she works with the intangible network of intelligent forces on behalf of her healing partner in need. I offer here some attempts to answer for myself that question of how did I get here, both in my own centering and in the TT interaction.

How Did I Get Here?—Centering

- I went to a "place"—a nonphysical dimension, a state of consciousness that is the stuff of dreams; that is, it was similar but not quite the same.
- I simply stepped out of my body and into the surrounding subtle-energy field, and in doing so it immediately felt like déjà vu.
- It was a timeless moment.
- I was aware only of quietude, peace, tranquility, even serenity. It was a friendly silence; nevertheless, it was permeated with a charged stillness.

How Did I Get Here?—The TT Interaction

- As I turn my attention to my client, my respiratory rate becomes slower and deeper, a profound "listening" state is available, and I notice that my hand and heart chakras have "turned on." I can still see as I normally do; however, my visual field seems to have shifted focus and I seem to be shortsighted, the focal point somewhere behind my physical eyes, while simultaneously my sight is coming from an area about two to three inches in front of the midpoint of my forehead.

- A strong bond of compassion links me to the patient and I am aware that my crown and *ajna* chakras are functioning. It is out of this compendium of subtle functions that I know where to lightly place my hand chakras on, or just beyond the periphery of, the patient's physical body as I continue the Therapeutic Touch healing session.

- I experience the power of focused mind-to-mind communion that elicits deep within me an intuitive grasp of the root of the problem, and a sensed, fleeting recognition, or a hint of a deep remembrance, or recall of the presence of an old, wise friend, an irreplaceable ally.

Various Healers' Personal Experiences of Major Assumption #4

- I sense and feel helpers on many occasions without calling on them directly. They are already helping guide the process.

- Sometimes I get a visitor, one of the angels or a deceased relative of the healing partner. For example, one healee's son suicided and after two years she had not recovered. While doing TT sessions and at times before or after, I get messages from her son. He says he is concerned about her. I pass this on, as this client is also a TT person. Using this as an example, I may be relaxing, preparing for bed, and I feel a presence. Then there is the mind-to-mind communication about the patient. This person's son again visits me and asks me to do more TT and support his mom.

- One experience I had that was really rewarding was with a man who was dying. I had never met him before the session, but he was so open and thankful. He was very cachectic and between worlds.

During the session two things happened. There was a silent communication that his wife could not let him go and this was holding him back. He was ready. He also asked me to do TT with his wife. I did so. I told his wife he was not able to go until she was able to let him. She was upset to see him suffer and did not want him to suffer any more. I suggested she might tell him it is okay for him to go and that she will be okay. Two days later I was exercising on my stationary bike when all of a sudden he was in the room with me. He had crossed and wanted to thank me for helping his wife. This was between 4:30 and 5 p.m. I received a call the next day from their friend who said he'd died the previous day at 4:30.

- In the approach phase I sometimes experience my guides helping me, and this was one of those times. I centered and had the psychic equivalent of bumping into a good friend in a crowd: "Oh, you're my partner today."

- Rebalancing: I have a fond memory of being at Camp Indralaya the last morning with some friends I had made down on Far East Beach. The sun was shining warmly and brightly down on us. I used that image and experience of feeling replenished gently by the warm sun while lying back on a warm rock with the peace of the ocean in the background. I have the energy of that memory ready at my left palm as a mist to be pulled in by the client's adrenals. I do this until the pulling slows or stops.

- Rebalancing: Smooth, tight areas, ask the healing partner to take deep breaths; clear areas. Hands on, hands off. I send calm, peaceful energy. I see the area as whole and balanced. Sometimes I call in helpers. Sometimes I sense them without calling on them.

- During rebalancing the energy is flowing through my heart center. I am guided through my third eye and crown chakra as well as heart. I am connected with the healee, Inner Self to Inner Self, and get messages that I follow. I send calm, peaceful energy. I use colors as needed, as well as metaphors as guided by my Inner Self. I see the area as balanced and whole as well as thinking of the person as whole. If I am feeling any resistance, or there is a lot to handle with respect to the individual's healing fields, I call on helpers. I get a sense or intuit who to call. Often it is Mother Mary and angels for whatever the need. For example, I will call on the person's guardian angel for help and perhaps an angel who is for healing or one for love. I am often guided by the crown chakra and the knowing of a person, and would call on Christ if guided to do so.

There is an understanding in Therapeutic Touch—one of our guiding principles—that there is an unlimited source of healing energy available to living beings. As Dora wrote: "There is a universal healing field in our cosmos; this seems to be the case since all living organisms have the capacity to heal themselves, and, under the appropriate circumstances, to heal others also. The two main components of the field are order and compassion."*

This understanding touches on one of the most basic differences between Therapeutic Touch and faith-based practices of laying on of hands. In the traditional rituals there was an understanding of a higher power who had selected the "healer" as a specially gifted person. Both the healer and the person in need shared the belief in that higher power. In Therapeutic Touch the qualities, the characteristics, the name of the energy of the universal field, all originate from the "within" experience of each individual healer. The healee does not have to subscribe to any view about the source of healing energies. Major Assumption #4 touches on ways that some TT therapists and some healing partners experience the healing energies. As we have shown, it is a common experience; however, it is in no way prescriptive.

---

*Dora Kunz, *Spiritual Aspect of the Healing Arts* (Wheaton, Ill.: Quest Books, 1985), 27.

PART 2

EXPERIENTIAL KNOWLEDGE OF HEALING

Therapeutic Touch
Exploratory Studies

6

"Looking Over My Shoulder," A Study in Mindfulness

There is an unmistakable personal knowing that the healer experiences during the TT session that sensitively guides her through subtle-energy patterns, organizes the bases of her decision-making, and structures significant questions about the ongoing healing interaction. However, these knowings occur in the moment and are very difficult to translate accurately into common language. Heretofore, aside from personally informed and acutely perceptive poetry, highly sensitive prose, and instrumental music, the experience has remained largely ineffable. In an attempt to cross this finely meshed psychic bridge we will begin by focusing on first-person accounts of TT therapists' experiences to see if we can catch a hint of what is transpiring in this profound, subtle encounter that occurs in the territory of the Inner Self.

The present study asks:

- What are the fundamental experiences during the processing of healing energies, as perceived through the practice of the Therapeutic Touch therapist?
- What does it feel like to be a sustained, living center for fine, vital life-energy flows running through your being?
- How can we define the lived experience of therapeutically oriented

subtle-energy surges that are guided by a deep-seated intentionality for the well-being of another?

To get a footing into the living bedrock of those events that support healing, an exploratory but penetrating examination of the interiorized expressions of the Therapeutic Touch therapist has formed the matrix of the present study.

Certain generalities occur. Nurse healers and, in fact, most clinicians use the experiences of their earlier professional preparation as the immediate base for making their physical assessments of the healing partner. Years of study of living pattern recognition have formed the basis of their realization of the classical diagnostic categories into which the symptoms of their various patients separate themselves. Since in the practice of Therapeutic Touch we are trained that our energy assessments are not intended to be congruent with a medical diagnosis, the TT therapist has learned to suspend these judgments as she and her patient enter the healing phase. It is essential to realize that in Therapeutic Touch we do not formulate any protocols based on the patient's diagnosis. Each session of TT is played out in the present moment; each TT therapist is present to her patient in that moment. She does not deny a diagnosis, but she remains present to whatever that patient presents *in that moment.* So often we hear a healer report something like: "The diagnosis was [x or y or z] but today what came up for the patient was a worry about a family member."

A TT therapist uses her perceptions to note any changes or dysrhythmias in the fine-energy flows of the healing partner over the duration of the treatment. She also observes both physical and emotional movement to capture the gestalt of the healing partner as cues to the ongoing subtle-energy dynamics. Along with any intuitive impressions, she notes information she receives from the movements of her hands through the pranic flow of the subtle energies of the healing partner; she then uses that amalgam of subtle-energy-patterned streaming as her perspective for assessing the whole array of clinical problems.

Therapeutic Touch therapists' resources include the use of the voice to explain and answer questions, and to pitch the tone of their voice to calm and to reassure. They may ask explicit permission to proceed to treat, unless the healing partner has come with that intent and the permission can be assumed. The TT therapist listens with her physical sense organs to the quality of the patient's voice to note vitality and affect. She may feel keenly an increasing intimate connection with him through her hands, her heart, her third eye, and her intuition. This sympathetic response to the individual's problems can sometimes be felt as physical discomfort. The therapist needs to stay mindful to remain centered in the impersonal space, so that she does not over-identify with the healing partner's symptoms and thus become part of the problem.

The therapist often puts her hands on the healing partner's shoulders to get a sense of his pranic flows, which converge in the area of the brachial plexus, the physical site of the anatomical "stress pool." She lends her own centered, healthy subtle-energy fields to the client as a scaffolding, which he can use as a healthy model in the repatterning of his own energy fields and work with them. As the therapist continues with the TT session she increasingly feels the effects of the fresh pranic flow surging through her, as she acts as a conduit for the healing partner's wellbeing. She also becomes sensitive to his readiness to receive treatment, often indicated by his taking a deep breath, an early sign of a profound relaxation response that typically follows as the TT session continues.

Simultaneously, the therapist becomes aware of her own inner signals of readiness—perhaps a sense of "tingling" in her hands, "heat" in her palms, and a surge of compassionate feeling arcing from her heart chakra to his heart chakra. Intuitive flashes about his condition may be sensitized by these strong responses of the heart chakra, and the aware therapist uses those intuitions to gain insight into physical and emotional issues of the healing partner. At the same time, she often intuits subtle hints about how to treat them. And so, one realizes, Therapeutic Touch is a path of continual and deepening learnings about the healing partner and, simultaneously, about herself as she treads this multidimensional pathway of compassionate concern for those who are ill, in trauma, wounded, or nearing final transition. This happens within the context of continued exploration of her own inner journey.

The Dual Aspects of Therapeutic Touch

Experiential

Dora Kunz and I always told our students to take nothing we told them on faith but to test out their own experiences in what we came to call the Laboratory of the Self. The heart of TT is the state of sustained centering. The TT therapist learns that not only does centering act as an empowering agent for healing others, it also provides a connection to her Inner Self. She learns that the compassion she feels toward the patient is an ally on her healing path.

As she stays on center during the TT assessment, she discovers a pattern of constellations of vital-energy flows, psychodynamic motifs, thought forms, and other expressions of consciousness. During the assessment she develops the sensitivity of her hand chakras in picking up these patterns as cues. Further, the relationship of the hand chakras to the heart and crown chakras empowers the therapist in her intention to help or heal. She may come to realize that visualizations are originating in the brow chakra, which then stimulates mind-to-mind communication via the crown chakra, which synergistically affects the entire chakra complex. As the therapist decides to direct energy from the universal field toward the patient, she remains grounded and centered; with intentionality she focuses the precise direction and depth of the energy offered to the patient.

Theoretical

From the time of the call from a person in need, the TT therapist feels compassion originating from the heart chakra, which becomes a power facilitating the TT process itself. She enters the state of sustained centering, an act of interiority. In this realm the therapist can learn to understand the dynamics of the vital-energy field without the use of contact/touch. Intentionality guides the decisions the therapist makes and becomes one of the signature powers of self. In the dynamics of the TT interaction, one may gain an understanding of the chakras as centers of different kinds of consciousness. The therapist senses cues from the vital-energy field of the patient as a way of receiving information.

This information can then be transmitted to other TT therapists.

"'Looking Over My Shoulder,' A Study in Mindfulness" is an initial query into healing, this most humane of all human quests, from the point of view of the healer.

The Purpose of the Study

The purpose of "Looking Over My Shoulder" is to assist the individual TT therapist to bring unconscious content and experiential knowledge into self-awareness. The phrase "looking over my shoulder" is used to mean "I stand behind myself and observe myself giving a TT session."

Therapeutic Touch provides an opportunity to awaken the deeper levels of the therapist's unconscious. TT accesses the subliminal area of the brain and extends to the nearer reaches of the Inner Self. This is where universal archetypal themes interact with the collective unconscious as the TT therapist engages the process on behalf of her healing partner.

The Practice of Therapeutic Touch

The practice of Therapeutic Touch provides an open sesame to a reality other than that of our everyday awareness, one that simultaneously operates on several levels of consciousness. The TT therapist uses the power of her compassionate yearning to access her energy flows (prana) in the multitasked charge to help or heal her healing partner, who is in an imbalanced state of pranic flow. Primarily the TT therapist acts to help his subtle-energy systems return to a more balanced state. She acts in the moment, mindful of her interior promptings, engaged in deep listening, to catch the intuitive guidance from her Inner Self as she helps or facilitates healing for another person with appropriate TT techniques. Meanwhile, she embarks on a journey within to seek out her Inner Self to act as her ally, guide, and teacher in this act of compassionate concern.

Learning to hone this faculty for intuitive communion over time, the TT therapist, in a state of interiority, works in concert with her Inner Self toward goals of high reliability in actualizing her potential for self-awareness.

In brief, the progressive phases of the TT process she engages to help or to heal her healing partner are:

1. She senses a call to help someone who is ill, in trauma, wounded, or approaching end of life.
2. She shifts into an altered state as she assumes a sustained centering of her consciousness and remains in that state throughout the healing session.
3. Driven by compassionate concern for the healing partner, she seeks within for help and guidance from her Inner Self.
4. She may feel increased receptivity and responsiveness from her vital-energy and psychodynamic fields toward her Inner Self, the healing partner and his Inner Self, and other intelligences.
5. As she continues her TT practice, she may become increasingly aware of a progressive and extended sensitivity that includes the sense that her upper chakras are "turned on" and fully alert.

Methodology

Prerequisites and sample size: To assure maturity of response, the participating TT therapists were required to have had at least three years' experience with the Therapeutic Touch process. There were twenty-eight participants in this study.

Scope of the Study

Although the TT experience during the healing session is a process and as such should be treated as a continuum, for the purpose of clearly articulating the scope of this study, the experience of a Therapeutic Touch session has been broken down into six succinct phases. Specific questions that defined each phase were asked of the participating TT therapists.

1. Call/Approach/Centering
What is your initial experience as you approach your healing partner (healee, patient, or client) at the beginning of each TT session?

2. Outreach

What are your hand chakras doing during the outreach phase as you reach for your healing partner and prepare to get into the TT assessment of his condition?

3. Search/Assessment

How are you picking up information? What chakras are activating? Is there a sequence? Can you describe it?

4. Rebalance

How do you know when your state of consciousness shifts? Do you use certain chakras? Do you hold your body in certain positions or postures? How do you assist your healing partner to shift into rebalance? What is the rebalancing that holds the most clarity for you?

5. Done

How do you know that the TT treatment is complete?

6. Recall

Do you have dreams, reveries, or any manner of interaction at a distance with your healing partner after the TT session? Which and how often?

As one participant wisely wrote, "It is hard to break into parts and pieces what is a natural ebb and flow of a healing and helping act, which comes from one's deep within and without—with the deep within and without of another. With TT one connects one's deep within of being to the deep within of another's being. The healing act has begun. The inner and outer are one with the universe. Invisible with invisible, but all seeing."

TT practice is primarily a right-brain experience. In early days of learning, a student's left brain will often object to the idea that anything could be happening in these invisible realms. Part of our development as healers is training the left brain to validate the right brain's perceptions.

Thus, our study, "Looking Over My Shoulder."

Responses to the Phases

Practitioners were asked to describe their response to the various phases of a healing session.

Approach Phase

To appreciate the fullness of the TT healing experience, responses were looked at from several perspectives during the TT approach. It is to be noted below that some therapists interfaced other therapeutic practices with definitive TT techniques, if that action was within the context of the healing partner's needs. This is within the broad definition of Therapeutic Touch practice.

Experiences with Similarities to Other Healing Modalities

Fifty-three percent began by doing some kind of physical evaluation of the healing partner, either an actual physical assessment or breathing in sync with the recipient in the approach phase.

Early in the approach the therapist often had mixed feelings that spawned a sense of apprehension, got caught up in the excitement of a new venture that was spurred on by anticipation of, and curiosity about, what was about to transpire, or felt low-grade anxiety: *What is the purpose of this healing session?* and *Am I good enough?* In this the therapist spoke to her own Inner Self questioning how to proceed, or often, feeling the presence of her Inner Self, remembering that *This is not about me,* and realizing *I am open to discovery,* accepting the healing encounter itself.

Twenty-eight percent of the group included personal practices, such as getting in touch with nature, self-quieting, preparing psychologically and spiritually to intercede for the healing partner, accessing the crown chakra, and petitioning some power or energy to help others. Several others silently asked the Inner Self of the healing partner for permission to heal, engaged in a personal ritual to open themselves to healing forces, or quietly intoned a repetitive call, saying, *peace* or *calm,* or actively projected toward the recipient saying, *I send my love and peace.* A few slowly approached the healing partner, mentally questioning: *Who is this being?*

Individual practices were prevalent, including prayer, intonations, mantras, and personal ritual. Several persons engaged in silent conversations with the Inner Self of the healing partner during the approach phase. Where appropriate, others explained TT to the recipient or used light humor; or played musical recordings as they approached. One therapist played the harp and another said, "*The Gayatri* [an ancient Sanskrit mantra] went through my mind."

Experiences Specific to Evoking the TT Process

Either before she begins the approach, during the approach, or as she reaches the healing partner the therapist accesses a sustained centering mode and continues in that alternative state of consciousness until the end of the session. Once firmly grounded in a state of sustained centering, the therapist begins the inner journey in quest of a connection with her Inner Self.

A prime factor underlying the therapist's engagement in the approach is a compassionate response to the call from someone in need. Once initiated, compassion acts as a psychic engine to drive the TT therapist's efforts during the healing session. The power of compassion supports the healer's continuing engagement to help or to heal the healing partner, and quickens the whole process.

The therapist begins the assessment, often placing her hands on the shoulders of the recipient, at the brachial plexus at the base of the back of the neck, or possibly over the adrenal area. In addition to activating the hand chakras while exploring the partner's subtle fields for signs of pranic imbalances, several TT therapists feel they are activating their third eye, the ajna chakra. Some feel they have engaged in vivid visualization of the problem areas. A few intentionally initiate the Deep Dee encounter, describing it as: "I am aware of an immediate engagement of my heart chakra with the partner's heart chakra," or, "I connect with the partner, Inner Self to Inner Self."

Experiences that Evoke Emerging Concepts

As the therapist continues she begins to sense an engaged presence. She learns to quiet herself and becomes aware of her Inner Self as her ally during the session. "I connect with the golden light within" was expressed by one participant in the study. As sustained centering becomes a more frequent behavior, the therapist often seeks out that state and routinely focuses into her Inner Self as she approaches the healing partner. With surprising rapidity she realizes that she can be in direct communication with her Inner Self as the need arises.

She begins to be consciously aware of a felt shift in consciousness, interest, and expectations as this direct relationship with her Inner Self continues. Her behavior changes in response and she finds that in the approach phase her actions are gentle; she speaks softly to her healing partner, who is now truly a partner or collaborator in this healing act. This deeply affects both therapist and recipient, and the therapist becomes increasingly aware that "there is a profound stillness" enveloping her and her partner. "The stillness," she says, "is a marker for my readiness." As she consciously deepens her experience with further practice, her comment now is: "I feel a shared connection in this silent space," and, "It is still and it 'feels' real." She has heard the "native language" of her Inner Self and it reinterprets the stillness for her.

Over time the therapist feels an increased awareness of her own energy fields. Concomitant with this, she is also more in communion with nature. Several persons noted that now "I get more intimately in touch with nature." She picks up cues of imbalance in the healing partner more readily with her hand chakras. Some TT therapists feel cues kinesthetically, while others could not distinguish the pranic flows as cues; that is, while they could not sort out the subtle-energy flows specifically, they could "feel" the healing partner's energy. Some therapists could clearly visualize their partners' subtle fields. The acuity ranged from "I noticed that internal stuff is bothering her" to "There was an immediate recognition of hidden issues in a partner's field," to comments such as "Encounters are slightly different in dealing with new healing partners; long-standing, familiar partners; and healing at-a-distance."

As the therapist gets more deeply into TT practice, there may be several indications that she is actively, consciously using her chakras. For example, "There is an instantaneous chakra involvement . . . as soon as I have the intention to work with a client." More specifically, "Almost immediately I get information about psychodynamic field interactions through my hand chakras," which is sent (made intelligible) by the heart chakra and the third eye. The hand chakras may become warm as the therapist maintains and deepens sustained centering. Others actually "feel the hand chakras being lighted up." With continued practice the therapist began "using my chakras as instruments." Another felt her "hand chakras open and be receptive, as if they were antennae." These practices took little effort: "My hands are gentle and moving," and, "I listen to messages [about my partner's condition] from my hand chakras," and could be highly specific: "My hand chakras were in both the here-and-now and at-a-distance realities."

The hand chakras seem to have the potential to perceive others' states of imbalance, as has been recorded since antiquity. Moreover, the hand chakras seem to be "pulled" to do the TT assessment, and begin to facilitate the helping/healing process. Says one therapist: "The hand chakras are tingling and drawn to get ready—they vibrate and there is a 'pull' to do a TT assessment on the healing partner." This pull is described as an attracting force that "pulls down," and, "the pulling is often like magnets."

To a third therapist, "My hands move through vibrations of the partner, assessing the temperature and density changes. During these times," she continues, "I often close my eyes and see . . . some color changes." Another responds to "slight tingles in the hands, and I get a blue-white color in my mind." Other responses include:

- I deep-listen to my hand chakras, getting (distinct) messages from my Inner Self's voice.
- Each hand is giving me different information and a synthesis has to take place to make the message understandable.
- [In reference to her hand chakras:] Several things are going on at the same time.
- I am always aware of my connection to Inner Self; it's like a continuous intelligent flow of energy to my hand chakras.

Two of the therapists attributed almost identical imagery to the hand chakras. One person described this as: "My hand chakras are like little cups that are (sensitive) to any changes." The second said, "Little ears connect my third eye and my heart chakras, then the energy goes down and grounds."

Other chakras seem to come under the therapist's control. The brow chakra (third eye) is next-most often mentioned. One therapist is able to access her brow chakra and note its functioning. Several others simply feel their brow chakras, and another states: "[With] my hand on the partner's sides, my third eye assesses [the rest of his body] . . . while our Inner Selves are connected. Messages come mostly from the heart chakra and are connected to the right-hand chakra, as the left hand very lightly and slowly assesses the healing partner from head to toe. I use the brow and crown chakras and also information from my fingers where they touch the recipient's fingers."

One of the most interesting of the Emerging Concepts is that of the therapist's development of the self-awakening of inner faculties as she moves more deeply into an understanding of her TT practice and her linkage with Inner Self. An early step occurs as the therapist's insight leads her to realize that for both herself and her partner, most of the vital aspects of the TT interaction take place in a "nonordinary" state of consciousness, the transpersonal.

As one healer stated: "Suddenly you realize you are standing outside of yourself . . . in a new space." Another indicator of self-awakening is the realization of having accepted a path of compassionate concern for someone in pain, trauma, illness, or in the process of final transition. Describing this realization, one therapist said, "In spite of a personal antipathy, there was a welling up of compassion to help an ill person that was irresistible, and a flood of empathy engulfed me." Another described the moment as: "I felt the grief of the partner in my own throat chakra." This awakening of one's own subtle abilities is vivified for those who use reference to oneself as a standard against which they assess the healee during the TT assessment. This can come close to identification with the healing partner as the therapist "feels the healing partner's suffering," or his "gut feelings" become apparent to her. Identification with the healing partner is contraindicated during the TT session, and it is the sustained centering maintained by the therapist that protects both healer and healee. A therapist reported that she feels "a fullness in my heart chakra," or she feels "a (distinct) rhythm in my hands" and "a connection is immediate" with the healing partner at these times. "I feel fully present," reports another. "There is an increasing sense of unition," another says. And from another: "I experienced being in a familiar, comforting place."

These types of responses could be reflected by healers across a variety of disciplines, and are not limited to TT therapists.

Additional Responses

- I always feel for their suffering and want to help. This is different from feeling their suffering. I could easily go there but know that gets me off center, so that route has an automatic "closed" sign on it. I always have anxiety about if I'm up to the task, concurrent with relaxation and a spontaneous remembering that it generally works out well and I am only responsible for bringing my best to it. This part zips by and leaves as I take my first centering breath and connect with the person's field.

- When approaching the healee I am aware of a fullness in the heart chakra. I experience a profound sense of compassion beyond myself—a very familiar space, like an old friend. Very comforting. It fills my being.

- In thinking about my approach I am paying attention in a different way—looking over my shoulder. I am very aware that I receive lots of information as I approach my healing partner. I am very aware that I receive cues within a web of senses but not much kinesthetically. Yes, I can feel sensations within my being, and no, I am not caught in the Four Dragons of fantasy, wishful thinking, exaggeration, or impulse. I do not assume; I listen deeply and pay attention. I am at peace with this and open to whatever presents itself to me within this moment, this connection. I also know, looking over my shoulder, that my sustained centering is manifest as I experience the profound stillness I feel when I stand in the sunlight under a blue sky. It is a stillness in which I hear sounds and feel the earth rhythms. I am not sure if these are the best words but I realize that this is my cue that I am ready.

Editor's Note: How Important Are Chakras in the Practice of TT?

As noted in an earlier chapter, conscious awareness of the healer's own chakra complex, as described by some therapists, is not a requirement for learning and practicing Therapeutic Touch. The use of the hands to pick up energetic cues is one way of perceiving. Often as people are first learning to do TT they may report not feeling anything with their hands, yet the person receiving the healing is aware of changes in his energy, thoughts, feelings, and physical sensations. The awakening of inner facilities is one of the benefits that many discover through the practice of TT. We learn that our intuition has multiple ways of communicating to us. Visualizations might include words, impressions, pictures, colors, a sense of an area of the partner's body, levels of physical vitality/fatigue, or something else. Keep in mind that all who participated in this study had a minimum of three years' practice of Therapeutic Touch, and many had much more.

As we begin to see, when the Therapeutic Touch therapist undertakes to help or to heal those who are ill, traumatized, in a state of bioenergetic imbalance, or approaching end of life, she enters a nonordinary state of consciousness, facilitated by the practice of sustained centering. Through the continued experience of this altered state over time, the TT therapist often comes to feel that Therapeutic Touch is a function of her spirituality. That is to say, it is primarily a way of healing "other" while learning to self-awaken her individual higher functions. Equally, it is a way to practice inviting the Inner Self into her daily life.

Over time, as we delved more deeply into the experience of the Therapeutic Touch process, we found that these meaningful personal experiences are held so firmly in the unconscious that the therapist herself is often largely unaware of the profound effects these often-intimate healing experiences have on her own behavior patterns, as well as those of the healing partner.

One characteristic of the TT experience that seems to hold a key to the activation of these deep-seated facets of her essential nature is the invariable occurrence of a penetrating stillness that seems to envelop the enactment of Therapeutic Touch. This is seen most dramatically when a group is being taught TT, for as they begin the actual practice of the process with a partner, a pronounced stillness settles over the entire group. In our study this descent of a sense of quietude was commented upon by most of the participants. When read in context, their comments about the quality of this unruffled, poised stillness makes clear that it is the onset of that tranquil state of being that is a prime indicator of the presence of the therapist's Inner Self. This surround of quiet and stillness during the healing session is a distinctive motif of the Therapeutic Touch process.

A second impression is that every single TT treatment is a unique encounter, whether the two persons meet only once or twice or encounters take place over an extended period, in relation to:

- What the healing partner needs
- The TT therapist's goals based on perceptions during *this* session
- Her previous experience, learning habits, culture, personal rituals, and belief system

Another perception at this stage of the study, a sense shared by many TT therapists, is that space and time do not seem to have the same influence over the outcomes of the healing session as they do in most other human behaviors.

Outreach Phase

In the outreach phase the healer moves toward the healing partner and sensitizes herself to his presence as she continues to move in his direction. Typically she extends her hands as she reaches toward the partner's vital-energy field. The information she picks up is of a subtle nature, and to make sense of the experience she is often thrown back on the use of metaphor or analogy, visualization, symbol, or intuitive hunches. Whichever she chooses, her perceptions become a figurative representation of her reality of the moment; however, the experience itself remains difficult to fully describe.

Findings

- Everyone had a slightly different experience.
- Responses were based on self-interpretation, and perspectives were framed by their individual backgrounds.
- All had indications they were in an altered state of consciousness and were perceiving things introspectively.
- They felt that although what they were engaged in was largely invisible and nonmaterial, over time they often found the experience had a reality base. For instance, one participant was able to verify a cue feeling like "an electric quiver" in persons with multiple sclerosis; two therapists were able to quantify their perceptions as having three distinct factors; one participant could clearly differentiate everyday experiences from peak experiences.

What are your hand chakras doing during the outreach phase as you get into the TT assessment?

✐ They're like little ears that pop up and become very attuned to any changes or differences. They and my brain work to translate this input into pictures and impressions, often wordless. I still have to work out synthesizing the information when each hand is giving me very different information. I have to be careful to just assess because it's tempting to adjust something as I sense it is off balance. They connect with my heart chakra and third eye/crown and then that energy goes down and grounds. It is three processes. One is feeding information to me, the second optimizes my energy flow, and the third shifts my energy so I feel differences that translate into inferences about the healee's situation and needs.

⚬ It seems that the more I feel the field and stay off the body, the more I am able to pick up energetic nuances and vibrations that over time I have come to feel represent the presence of medication in the fields of certain people. At first it was very jittery, especially over and around the head. As time has gone on and the healing partner is less frightened of the medicine (and is understanding the importance of thoughts and how they affect the body), I can feel the medication throughout the field but it is more subtle, and less fear and anxiety are present in the field.

⚬ I am trying to resonate with the healee's field, which in turn may give me a picture of the problem. By attuning to the rate, rhythm, and vitality of the field and energy flow, I am able to conceptualize the imbalance. I can focus on the hand chakras but I seem to import information through intuition or through all my chakras. This process starts the "image" of the healing template, which is perceived at this juncture.

⚬ Each time I get a bit lost I relax back into my heart chakra and listen from there. But I have to let my heart chakra connect with that universal wisdom/intelligence—not my "idea" of universal wisdom or wholeness and order, not my definition, but the living experience.

⚬ My hands are very close to his field, especially in front of his legs. His field is close to his body and feels deflated. His field is thicker in the back. My hands are warm and tingly.

⚬ [In this session,] I enter and rest my hands on my partner's arm. My hands palpate the continued thickness and note the quality of her field. I feel the unevenness of her field around her chest, but I notice it has held and is fuller than yesterday. I work with the thin field adjacent to her leg.

⚬ My hand chakras first made a clear connection with the information-gathering channels of my mind, body, and energy field. Then they reached out to scan my partner's field in the prescribed manner. The chakras sensed some clear cues from the physical body in addition to those pertaining to the healee's complaints. There was also a disturbing feeling/sense that serious imbalances were present in both the physical and mental/emotional areas that had not been offered during the initial conversation. The awareness surfaced here that an Inner Self–to–Inner Self connection would be required to understand the mental/emotional imbalances, if that were acceptable to the healee's Inner Self.

🖉 As I reflect on my hands I realize that my outreach is a deepening of connection. I use my hands in the way that appears to be the right way and I sense what this way is . . . whether holding hands or whatever. I do start treatments—most of the time—in the back by gently touching the healing partner's shoulders, and then touch both my heart and the partner's shoulder. I also realize that I am not talking about a habit pattern. I adapt my outreach as I believe is indicated with each individual session. This looking over my shoulder is really quite the fascinating experience. I am deeply exploring my practice.

Search/Assessment Phase

Continuing on her healing journey, the TT therapist now metaphorically "crosses the bridge"; that is, she turns her full attention to the search and steps with confidence into a new dimension of perception.

TT therapists begin the session by gathering bits of subtle information about the healing partner's state of being during the search/assessment of the partner's subtle-energy (pranic) flows. In this phase we take a cue from the age-old tradition of perceiving healthy vital-energy systems as being "in balance" with each other, and "in a state of imbalance" when they are unhealthy. It is during this search that the healer tests the healee's various energetic complexes for their current state of balance or harmony. This fundamental exploration includes the study of the vibratory and flow patterns, rhythms, and the state of being of the healer's subtle energies. After these several factors have been evaluated, the therapist then decides how best to assist the partner to rebalance his total energetic being at whatever level seems appropriate, or to the extent that his field allows at that time.

The responses in this section speak to the simultaneity of the TT process. During the formal teaching, when people are new to the process, it is helpful to delineate the phases as actual steps, to allow a linear understanding for the purpose of learning. Eventually we find that beginners naturally evolve into more of a simultaneous relationship among the phases as they become more comfortable in their practice.

This realization by one participant as she worked with the healee speaks to the presence of natural human potential and how the practice of TT leads therapists into deeper levels of self-awareness: "I began to really put things together with these questions. I realized that ever since I was a little girl, my solar plexus and third eye have worked together to observe and assess a person. It was a protective mechanism; I grew up in a situation where I was vulnerable and found this was helpful in my life. When I went into nursing it was natural to assess the patient and go beyond just the physical.

"One example of how it worked for me before TT was as a new R.N. I was night-charge nurse on a Med Surg floor [for care of patients with medical or surgical complications]. We had a patient who was a large man. He was very loud and abusive to staff. One evening he was standing naked in his room, cursing out the aides and orderly. Everyone was scared of him. I went to the door and my physical eye, plus my solar plexus, assessed the situation. I did not see a naked man. My third eye communicated that I was seeing a scared little boy and between my solar plexus and third eye, they communicated with his heart. I was told—an inner voice?—that he was safe to approach but that he needed/wanted to have me approach him and communicate with him, and I did. I approached him sending love and peace. I asked what he needed and talked with him. He calmed down and he seemed to know it. This is how I often start to connect with a healing partner."

Other responses from various study participants regarding the search/assessment phase included:

- Listening with hands, watching, and watching with hands. Sometimes I feel that I'm also doing this with my chakras.
- Checking for balance—places that just don't feel right during the assessment, and often I feel these imbalances in my own body.
- Visually, as in third eye, and sensing as in heart connection.

Sensations are also felt in the hands, as pin sticks or coolness.

- My hand chakras are coming more alive as I get into the search/assessment. It happens when I am centered and I enter the vital-energy field of the healing partner. I have a vibratory sense in my palms that changes as my hand chakras sense the vital-energy and psychodynamic fields. Over the years they have guided me in my TT treatments and helped me become more discriminate with both assessment and treatment.

- My hand chakras are transmitting some of the information for me, but also my entire field picks up information. I am aware of my emotions feeling my partner's emotions; my mind feeling her state of mind. I am also aware of her patterns of stress and her nervous system. I don't understand it all yet, but I'm getting this information and also letting myself consciously and purposefully open to her and her information. I am also aware of really grounding myself and breathing slowly and deeply to be quiet, to center in that inner place of quiet so that I can listen.

- There are layers of information. On the surface I think the sensations I feel relate to pain, poor circulation—the physical functioning of her body. There is something in the upper back, something cool around the feet, something huge in her head. As I work through these requests for shifts, another layer is exposed and here I think I am beginning to touch the emotions that underlie the physical expression. I work as before, from head to toe, but allow myself to enter a deeper connection with the cues and work from the front to address a disturbance on her back. The emotional field seems able to receive (pranic flow) more directly. Is there a sequence? I suppose the sequence is physical, emotional, etheric. The final round of TT is where I ask her ancestors to continue to work with her, and my hands are moving to encourage and support, rather than shift any energies.

- My hands pick up her thin, irritable field. I am moving from my mental God-only-knows stance to calm, heartful attention, moving within the field in her chest torso, with intentions of helpful support over her adrenals. I use my inner eye (sixth chakra) to look at her heart. As she is relaxing, I am also relaxing, calm in knowing that our Inner Selves are connecting and good things are happening. With my hand chakras I am feeling her field fill in and flow to her feet.

🖉 The information doesn't come all at once. There seems to be an initial gathering of information that gives me enough to have an overall picture, but also a place from which to start the rebalancing. But as the treatment continues, and the more the "surface" cues are rebalanced, then I find myself searching once again with my hand chakras, probing her field, and from my Inner Self I hear, *What else?* This is when I find the deeper imbalances of dysrhythmia within her chakra system, and especially how her nervous system's habit pattern of disrupting her digestion comes to light. Again, it is listening from my Inner Self (heart chakra); and my hands are passing through her field and that information is then transmitted through my chakra system . . . and I am listening from that living experience of natural order that I can connect to/through my Inner Self.

🖉 My hands felt warm as I did a quick TT assessment (search) from the side and noticed that her field was very constricted. As she let me in, or as I grounded more fully, I noticed that she had hot inflammatory puffiness along her left sciatic nerve in the distribution of her pain and in the area she had described as puffy. My left-hand chakra stroked this area ("unruffled") to move the excess "hot stuff" down her leg to her foot.

🖉 I feel uncomfortable comparing my chakras to the healing partner. I feel I am too sensitive, or not clear enough within myself to not lose myself in my partner when comparing. What especially seems important to me is that during the entire time I am scanning, a part of me is relaxing into that living energy of wholeness, order, and compassion (universal life-energy) and I am doing this through and with my Inner Self. This being in a different consciousness really makes a huge difference. Before I had to imagine order, wholeness, and so on. Now—and this is largely due to my devic-consciousness explorations in nature—I relax into a vibrant living consciousness. I've learned to take my time, to wait for the inner process to take place. Listen, listen, listen and then let the information run though the intelligence of my chakra system, my current levels of consciousness within my chakras. This will show me. It feels that I have entered into a whole new world with TT now. I feel that I can actually treat people now, where before I was using Band-Aids.

🖉 I continued to center and to connect with her heart chakra. She ceased talking and fell into a reverie, as did I. Her husband remained silently supportive from across the room. She took a deep breath and relaxed under my hands. I put them physically against her low back and intended support. I put my hands over her adrenal glands at her back. I assessed her field and felt it thin and irregular, uneven. There was an irritable quality to it. My mind assessed this odd quality as the effects of the adrenaline (which had been medically administered for allergies). I moved my hands through the field around her face, intending the red puffiness to subside.

🖉 Although the vibratory sense in my hand chakras is my primary mode of sensing, I often get variations of heat or cold as well. With this healing partner I did get different levels of intense heat as I treated her neck. This indicated to me a change in the amount of congestion from the surgical site and the appliance in her neck. I also sensed a different level of heat coming from her wrists, hands, ankles, and feet. It felt less intense but somehow deeper, and it also encircled joints and appendages, as if holding them energetically.

The healer moves more decisively into the healee's personal territory, his vital-energy and psychodynamic fields, as she begins to focus more deeply in the search/assessment phase. Concomitantly, she continues to sustain a centered state of consciousness, a medium that is a favorably conducive atmosphere for the presence of Inner Self. It is of keen interest to note that now, when she is in the throes of helping or healing someone else, she has an exceptional opportunity to consciously and closely ally herself with her own Inner Self and, through that experience, to better understand the "native tongue" of her inner guide and ally.

As the identification with Inner Self deepens, so does the healer's concern for the well-being of her healing partner. Questions arise: *Who is this person I am healing?* is often the unspoken query as she focuses in on cues, energy-based indications of something that is amiss, or systems of prana that no longer flow, but are congested so that a blockage has occurred and normal flow is now in gridlock. Or the cue may be felt as a sense of heat or cold that does not translate to temperature in the physical sense; that is, for instance in the case of heat, the sense of it is not as would be the case as when approaching a flaming candle. The "heat" felt by the TT therapist is not in the cutaneous tissues, as would ordinarily be the case, but as energy or an intuitive knowing.

Some further responses to search/assessment in our study revealed more specific types of exploration:

- I use my hands as scanners, and that opens access to the information. I first attend to those cues and then realize that my head, especially the ears and sometime the rest of the body, especially the throat, are feeling changes in pressure. It is very important that I detach from interpreting it or translating it into images. If I do that, I lose data and am less attuned when I go from assessment into rebalance.

- The challenge is tracking and synthesizing multiple streams of information without moving into analytical mode. Breath helps, breath that goes from my lungs down my legs. If I get it down there, the breath automatically circulates to the rest of my body. I will admit that sometimes I don't get much information on the first pass and have to trust that more will be received. Then I start facilitating the prana flow with my hands from the top down, which allows the field to reveal itself to me as it starts to shift. And/or I do a hands-on movement of prana down the healee's back.

- Re: What chakras are kicking in? At this point in my development that question makes me think too much, and overthinking is my nemesis. I know I use my hand chakras and my breath in a way that can involve any of the chakras. I notice that I use my solar plexus and breath to help me stabilize. When I connect deeply to my source through my heart chakra, I get my best information.

- Re: Is there a sequence? I offer this tentatively. Centering helps all my central chakras to connect. It especially helps me connect heart and third eye chakras, and when all of the central chakras connect, this involves my hand chakras.

🖉 My hand chakras are picking up the quality of his deflated field. My heart chakra is sending him compassion, well-being, and care, and feeling his sadness, loneliness, and discouragement.

🖉 I start with hands on her shoulders and center my consciousness. I notice that I am slower or she is resistant to my "feeling" her field. It takes a bit for us to join our Inner Selves. I have access only to the front of her body, as she is in a chair and I do not ask her to move her body, but access her there, eventually sitting on the floor myself. I feel how close to her body she holds her field and how shallowly she breathes. Her relaxation is barely perceptible. She moves very little during our session. I intend through my heart and feel her field fill and become "fat." I use my hands on her legs to help move the flow down. I look with soft eyes and sixth chakra at her heart area. My mind is surprised at how brightly it sparkles and how lovely the golden light sparks from her center.

It is very interesting to note that there are several factors apparent during the Therapeutic Touch session and its sequelae that are not readily perceived in everyday life. Of prime significance is the stillness that descends on those involved in the TT session—as has been mentioned. This stillness occurs with dependable regularity and is noticeable by the time the search phase begins, continuing to be perceived until the end of the session. The presence of stillness is so common that it becomes a motif of the practice. The stillness is accompanied by a physiological relaxation response in the recipient, which, in controlled studies, has been found to occur within the first four minutes of the beginning of the TT session and to continue throughout the session and sometimes after it is over.

As was mentioned, the effects of Therapeutic Touch treatment do not seem particularly relevant to the bounds of space-time as we know it; a sense of timelessness, in fact, is one of the reliable constant experiences during TT sessions. Changes may continue to happen to the recipient for some time after the session is over, when the healing partner is no longer in the presence or proximity of the therapist. Sometimes the therapist can visualize the healing partner when the two are some distance apart—and TT at this distance may be experienced, with verifiable therapeutic results. Also, during visualizations that may occur to the therapist during a treatment, she might be able to "see" the origin of that individual's problem, or other relevant previous occurrences or information.

Consistent TT practice over time seems to have a reliable crossover to the continued development of the higher cognitive abilities. There also seems to be an enhanced coherency in reference to abilities to organize musings and seemingly disparate ideas, and to clarify budding conceptual frameworks about the dynamics of healing itself.

Other, more sensitive facets of the healer's being come to the fore, such as intuition and clarity in perception. The involved TT therapist can, and frequently does, awaken to the subtle realities of nature and, over time, to its intelligences. She may come to potentiate latent psychic abilities, such as clairvoyance and mind-to-mind communication.

Rebalance Phase

In the rebalance phase the healer interacts very closely with the healee, in reference to the repatterning of dysrhythmic energy flows toward health and rebalance. During this therapeutic interaction the surrounding subtle-energy fields significantly affect the TT interaction, and the interaction affects the fields, in clear declaration of the intrinsic integrated holomovement that forms the subtle ground of this process.

As noted previously, a profound relaxation response is the prime reliable effect of Therapeutic Touch. The relaxation effect has been found to significantly facilitate the immune system; it stimulates the production of neuropeptides, called endorphins, which act to block pain. Because of this, after and frequently during a Therapeutic Touch session, both children and adults fall asleep. They tend to awaken refreshed and vitalized and at least momentarily reinvigorated.

In a further effort to understand the rebalance phase, a series of questions was posed to participants:

1. How do you know your consciousness shifts?
2. Do you use certain chakras?
3. Do you hold your body in certain positions or postures?
4. How do you assist your healing partner to shift into rebalance?
5. Describe a rebalancing experience that holds the most clarity for you.

How do you know your consciousness shifts?

- I feel the shift in my physical body, but also within my own field, which is not as defined as physical touch but more like a knowing and sensation.
- By experience and by losing awareness of the area outside of my and my healing partner's energy fields.
- I shift right away, and then go deeper during assessment into another state of being, interconnected with the healing partner. Key is to stay centered.
- When I shift into high gear and really get cooking, everything becomes crystal clear and shiny. I feel solid and whole and the world looks new, shiny, and friendly. I experience a sense of a flow that makes everything feel right.
- I can feel it and I almost lose my balance as I am standing there—as if walking into a new energy state.
- I'm not aware time has passed.
- I am aware of my field being centered and very present, energetically full, expansive, and embracing the healing partner in light.
- I sigh and sometimes I feel a river of relaxation moving down my body to my feet. Sometimes I have the psychic equivalent of feeling a lid snap into place. Usually I'm so absorbed in what I am doing that I don't notice until sometime after the fact.
- I refocused on the higher connection with my partner—and darned if his Inner Self didn't smile back.
- In the centering it is like the world quiets and I am only right here with the healing partner. The vibration around me becomes more pliable and I feel a connection with my Inner Self that almost feels like a voice, although it is not something I hear, but there is a presence that is different.

🖉 In reflection I am noticing two cues. One is an ever-deepening, profound stillness, a quiet that is really hard to describe. The healing partner and I are two but one, if that makes any sense. The other sensation is a lightening—it is still a quiet but it is lighter (the only word that comes to me).

Do you use certain chakras?

🖉 I send comfort and peace through hand and heart chakras, and sense a calmness within myself. I often sense a shift in myself (and my own chakras) where I think the shift has also occurred in the healing partner.

🖉 I know I use my hand chakras and my breath in a way that can involve any of the chakras. I notice I use my solar plexus and breath to help people stabilize. When I connect deeply to my source, through my heart chakra, I get my best information.

🖉 I intentionally engage my heart chakra as much as I can. My hand chakras normally become quite active during rebalancing. I do not focus on my healing partners' chakras as I believe this interferes too much with their healing processes. I prefer to pull, coax, or cajole their energy toward where it is needed, rather than push it there.

🖉 I follow guidance of third eye, heart, and solar plexus throughout and pick up messages intuitively both in ear and head. Sometimes I get a picture of the problem in my mind's eye and watch as it is rebalanced. Energy is flowing through heart center. I am guided by third eye and crown chakra as well as heart.

🖉 I think the hand chakras reach out instinctively and then, as the sensation of the field arrives, the heart and third eye kick in almost simultaneously. I am most aware of the solar plexus when I am moving my hand slowly, and my heart chakra when I am supporting the flow.

🖉 Energy flows down through my head and up through my feet to heart chakra and down my arms to my hand chakras; left for sending and right for rebalancing.

Do you hold your body in certain positions or postures?

Many said their own positions varied depending on that of the healing partner. Many also noted they tried to keep their spine straight or supported in some fashion. A few talked of integrating yoga or *qi gong* postures.

- For treating the healing partner in bed: To get her right side I actually lie on the bed beside her, and crawl on the bed as needed to get to all parts of her; and I also have her turn on her side so that I can assess and clear her back. She really likes touch on her back and then stroking from the top of her head down her spinal cord. For her it feels like a nice back rub, but my intention is to bathe the nervous system in healing energy—sometimes blue, sometimes clear—to help prevent any neuropathy from the chemo.

- It's the same way I hold myself when I stand and ready myself to do qi gong. Even when I bend, energy still runs through my body rooting me to the ground and keeping me connected to the sky. My movements are graceful and done with "ping," as one of my teachers would say, which means simultaneously focused and relaxed intention.

- I simply try to relax my body. When I withdraw to center into my deep center I often find that my hands (or one hand) are at my heart center—I just realized that! It is very helpful for me to sink into my feet physically. I'm learning t'ai chi right now and I find that it is helping me to sink into my feet more easily and feel supported physically from this.

- Generally my back is straight and I move up and down with my knees. The energy flows so much better through me that way; I am more open to receiving messages from chakra to chakra.

- It depends on the position of the client. I was able to kneel and work on a client lying on a couch using my left hand as the sender and the right as the rebalancer. I do my best to remain in healthy alignment for my spine at all times. However, I find that when I am leaning over someone and not able to kneel or stand straight, I get cramps in my low back and the flow diminishes from my heart to my hands.

How do you assist your healing partner to shift into rebalance?

- I wrap the partner energetically in love and peace, holding a vision of his wholeness. I do this with my entire field as I move my hands through his field to the areas that seem to need individual attention, as well as all areas of the body: head, shoulders, arms, back, legs, and feet, and often end with holding their heart area.

- I consciously use colors, images, emotions, and thoughts to promote rebalancing. By projecting a relaxed, caring attitude, I place myself just within the noticeable edge of the partner's energy field in a relaxed, open attitude but not close enough to generate a feeling of intrusion.

- I lightly caress the energy field three to four inches out from the healing partner and then "hold" his field for a little while.

- I'm aware of my breathing and the gradual mutual rhythm of our breathing.

- I silently express my intention to the healing partner and ask permission to help. I focus on my sense of humility before the greatness of the concept of helping another human to health, and on my sincere compassion for her. I won't claim that it is telepathy, but it seems to work.

- Reassessing from head to toe, sensing more areas that need to be rebalanced.

- I visualize her ankle in an unswollen, healthy state and silently ask the healing partner to do the same. I move hands down and away in a sweeping motion. I visualize "TT blue"* in and around her field, especially her ankle.

- Overall clearing, then work on his feet and smooth down his legs. I bathe the nervous system in healing (sometimes TT blue, sometimes clear light).

- I am at the healing partner's back, supporting his spine (chakras) while sending energy through the heart chakra, and modulating the rate and rhythm. While rebalancing, the image of the energetic template is held in my consciousness with the intention of actualization by the healing partner.

---

*See glossary entry for a description of TT blue. —*Editor*

- I usually clear the energy field, hold the feet to facilitate grounding for the partner, and move back to the head to reassess when rebalancing.

- I feel as though I can look into the body and see dense, thick energy like a thick tree branch and knot at the knee. It responds to a white star-like energy to release, then soothing blue-white energy.

- I flutter or quietly snap my fingers to assist in breaking up stagnant energy. I move my hands with sweeping motions away from the core, breathing with the moving—pushing away, then breathing to direct clean, healing energy.

- I send energy to her shoulders by first gently wrapping warmth around her. Then I send energy from my hands.

- I slightly close my eyes and concentrate on awareness of breath, if anything, during the treatment. My physical body is secondary to my awareness. During rebalancing I use visual images when the field is not moving easily. In this case an image is coming from the field that helped bring us together; nails rhythmically building a structure.

- Again, with breath. I find the partner's resonance, match it, and help it to move to a more balanced place. I may find myself making faster passes with my hands and then gradually slowing down, or the other way around. It's the way a good rider and horse work together as one unit. Using color doesn't come to me naturally, but I've been experimenting with it. Although I can't visualize it well in the healee, it is received just fine, as when I have projected TT deep blue and inflammation has receded. Otherwise I do what most people do: hands on, moving energy by working in one of the fields nearest the body, using my hand to project energy. Sometimes I like to have my hands doing one job while my mind (words fall short here) projects intuition somewhere else. I use my other chakras to hold the space. This isn't quite right; I haven't figured out how to put it into words. I don't have the luck some people have with seeing the healee whole and well or consciously connecting with the healee's Inner Self. My mind can get so easily caught up in thinking and ideas and chattering that these approaches distract me. I do best if I keep myself immersed in the sensory and intuitive cues I perceive. I believe I automatically connect with the healee's Inner Self.

- I feel in my being almost a "release." My intention is to offer quietness. With gentle, soft motions of my left hand while my right is on her left shoulder, I send quiet. I become aware of a beautiful light-creamy pink coloring that is enfolding. I am drawn to her solar plexus where I actually see a bright light that is not really colored. I know it is time to send energy to her adrenals. I am using hand motions and moving crown to foot in continuous sweeps that are ordered and rhythmic. I do not know for how many minutes this continues.

- By balancing and centering myself (scaffolding), I use this as a role model for the field of the healing partner to follow and balance.

- I get quieter inside as I assess the abdominal area. I can feel the nervous system alertness and "wound-upness," but in wanting to feel the layers of imbalance I get quieter within myself. I consciously relax more into my heart chakra and connect with my crown and with my Inner Self, and from there expand and come into harmony with universal order and wholeness. It is a different level of quietness and listening, as if I am listening from wholeness.

- I moved my hand downward along her left sciatic nerve path to rebalance the hot inflammatory stuff adjacent to her buttock and leg in the distribution of her pain pattern. She was standing and I stood alongside her. I knelt on the floor when I brought my hands to her feet to bring the energy down to ground. I assessed her field and found that the contour was fuller, even across her buttocks and legs. I "felt" with my hand chakra that her energy was flowing to her feet.

- Today it is that sense of compassion for his pain, and heart, and Inner Self connection within me and connecting to his Inner Self and to that universal healing energy through this connection that is foremost in my mind.

Describe a rebalancing experience that holds the most clarity for you.

- When I can feel a gentle push back from the field of the healing partner, it provides me with an indication of how much to send.

If this response from the partner gets stronger, I work more gently. Having this sense of where the healee is in the process and how it is going for that person gives me the most clarity.

- This is from a session with a person with cancer. Her energy felt cold, heavy, and dead. My mind started to worry about how to move it, wondering if I was doing it right and if it would move. I worked/non-worked to keep that energy flowing up and out, out of the way, while my more focused self listened deeply for what floated to the surface. Why things float up instead of down, I don't know. Sometimes they flow out of the body. In some ways "flow" describes it better than float. Float is part of it because it connotes a light, sometimes barely perceptible shift that may have spaces in it, while flow connotes a steady movement, in this case smooth and effortless. When an accurate direction hits me, I feel like Samantha's face on the old TV series *Bewitched* when she had an idea and was about to do a "witch" thing. It's an inner *oooo* of having the right move click in and being "happy" to implement it: nonverbal and often somatically experienced. It involves a sense of deep satisfaction. The *oooo* comes in after some time of deeply listening and heralds an influx of healthy energy into the stagnant area.

- Of course in the rebalancing there is continued assessment. I find that now I take my time and try to clue into the order in which I should unravel the imbalance(s). This order comes from my continued connection through my Inner Self to that universal healing energy comprised of order, wholeness, and compassion. I often feel that I am missing a piece of the picture, so I have learned to sit back into my heart chakra and listen again to the partner's field from that place of consciousness. I often remind myself of the "natural human potential for healing." If I focus on the energy of potential I am usually rewarded with an insight as to how to continue (even if the "continue" is to be finished because I have reached my limit or the partner has).

- I moved my hands to unruffle especially his lungs from the back. I put my hands over his adrenals and low back to support him. I allowed energy to flow between my hands into his chest. I felt his field expand. From his feet I saw that his heart was bright with light, but there was darkness in the center of it. My mind noticed that his field was responding to the TT and becoming fuller. It occurred to me that he had taken on a dark energy. I saw a dark something near his left shoulder and asked for help in making it leave if it was not for his highest good.

🖉 I moved my hands to a few inches away from her chest, intending to go all the way through and from my heart chakra. I moved my hands on her legs to draw the irritable energy down and to the ground. I looked up with soft eyes and saw a dark center in her heart with lots of light around it. The dark something jumped around, sometimes outside her body. (Later my mind said *abuse scar* on her heart; generous, engaging personality, and also genuine warmth.) I held my hands on either side of her heart and gradually her field filled and became more even. I noticed the flow of energy in her legs improved and her field fattened.

🖉 Working with his inflamed liver, feeling into the tissues, sending blue as I continue to feel into the tissues, to understand them; under the inflammation was an energetic connection to his heart chakra.

🖉 After treating the physical issues discussed in the initial conversation, I continued to work on what presented as congestion of the lungs. (A week later I was told that multiple spots on her lungs had disappeared in a follow-up medical scan.) The other item of concern was a hidden sadness and loss of interest in life and living. This was addressed with an overall flow of energy to my partner while maintaining Inner Self contact with the intent of concentrating on the value and goodness of personal and family/friends connections in physical life. (I later found out that she had lost a young son a few years prior.)

Odds of Success

It is impressive to consider the scope of dysfunctions that are sensitive to Therapeutic Touch, particularly considering that most TT interventions are based on experiential knowledge.

It has been well established that the physiological system most sensitive to TT is the autonomic nervous system, which suggests that the illnesses most responsive to TT are psychosomatic in origin. This is quite significant, for public health statistics report that at their inception, approximately 70 percent of illnesses in this stress-laden world are psychosomatic.

In my experience the systems that tie for second place in responsiveness to the TT process are the lymphatic and circulatory systems, and slightly behind them is the genito-urinary system. Additionally, I have found that gastrointestinal and musculoskeletal systems, particularly in the case of fractures, respond well to Therapeutic Touch treatment. Other nurses and laypeople may have different experiences.

All of the vital signs—internal body temperature, pulse readings, respiratory rate, blood pressure readings, and level of pain—are very sensitive to Therapeutic Touch. Swelling, wounds, blood disorders (particularly hemoglobin-based), fatigue, dizziness, shock, nausea and vomiting, apprehension, restlessness, anxiety, and fear seem to top the list of best reactions to TT treatment. In addition, there is a large spectrum of ills for which TT is notably effective, from the treatment of severe burns (particularly in the successful embedment of newly-seeded tissues), to the setting of musculoskeletal dislocations, done particularly by early responders in remote locations, ski patrols responding to accidents on the slopes, and firemen during emergencies. It is important to note that, even under circumstances when we cannot seem to eliminate symptoms of "dis-order" and "dis-ease," the relaxation response felt by the healee can still help. We always remember that TT is not about curing but rather the intrinsic movement toward order. TT has a long and highly reliable record of helping persons with terminal illness through the stages of their final transition and, where appropriate, TT easily adapts to interfacing with other healing methods.

As noted, patients frequently sleep during or after TT treatment, and often awaken with a sense of deep peace and well-being. This gives the sense that much that happens during the TT session occurs *sub rosa*—below the levels of perception of which we are normally aware—and that large amounts of that material are likely to remain a mystery for a considerable time, until our traditional ways of thinking radically change.

Experiential knowledge has become the healer's method of choice for gaining knowledge, largely because, outside of couching healing phenomena in a deeply faith-based orientation, there have been no adequate objective choices for teaching, learning, and explicating many of the strangenesses inherent in the healing way (happenings for which our culture has no logical frame of reference, such as when healing occurs without contactual touch, as it does with Therapeutic Touch). The therapist fosters her self-awareness so that she can become sensitive to changes that occur in her sensorium during the healing act. She also learns to recognize subtle changes occurring concurrently within the healing partner during the session, and uses these observations therapeutically during the rebalance phase.

These kinds of experiences make her cognizant of how intervention at one level of consciousness affects functioning at the physical level as well as the emotional, interpersonal, mental, and spiritual levels. While in this state of quietude and self-study, which is occurring simultaneously with the support she offers the healee, she perfects her ability to offer as a template the patterning of her own subtle energy in a technique called "scaffolding." This technique can reinforce the weakened field structure of the healing partner, through the principle of resonance. Dynamics of this rapport is analogous to what happens at the emotional level of consciousness when the therapist is in a state of compassion, as she is attracted to someone in need. As some of these participants have expressed, during the TT interaction she feels that she and the healing partner are at-one, and in the case of experiential knowledge, the knower and the known are closely bonded. In both cases, once the intent to act is focalized, the enactment of that intentionality is effortless, expressed by one therapist as "a calm and motionless sense of expansion."

Done Phase

Done, within the TT context, is not an absolute state. The state of the fields of the healing partner is relative to many things and "done" actually means done at this moment. One of the aspects of TT sessions we have learned is that the energy continues to integrate in the field of the healing partner after the formal session has ended. Sometimes in teaching we encourage students to end the session when the thought arises, "I wonder if we are done."

Usually before the therapist leaves the healing partner she does a reassessment to find out whether his condition has improved, whether she should recommend a referral to another therapist who may have other therapeutics to offer him, and how she might treat the partner the next time they meet, if TT sessions are to continue. Recognizing when a healee is done needs a fine sense of discrimination, for if she misses those signs and continues the treatment the healee may go into an energy overload. Consequently, the therapist stays aware of signs of restlessness, fatigue, pain, anxiety, or panic.

As Dora and I taught from the early days, it is better to underdo rather than overdo when it comes to sending energy. We can always come back and do more after a period of observation of how the healing energy is being assimilated by the healee's pranic systems. To help in assimilation, when the therapist determines that the healee is done, the usual procedure is to have the healing partner lie down for fifteen to twenty minutes to ground the energy, allowing time for integration.

TT therapists experience this shift in consciousness in a variety of ways:

- I know that the treatment is finished when my hands move through all areas of the healing partner's field in resonance with my own field. I get a deep sense of satisfaction and a sense that we have completed our "dance."
- In general, my attention disconnects. There's a sense that I've done enough for the time being. The energy flow is more even. My hands usually bounce (pulse) regularly. I just feel done.
- I receive the silent message that we are finished for the moment.
- When the moment begins to pass, I quickly smooth down, ground, smooth down, ground, brush down the healee's field, and disengage.
- It is an intuitive flash, a deep knowing. A knowing when the healing

partner needs to modulate the experience through the rate and rhythm of his energy field. A recognition/feeling of wholeness.

- I'm not sure *when* consciousness shifts, but I realize something happened when I'm done and I'm not aware of time passing.

- I usually draw to a close when I feel no more energy drawing from my hands.

- When I feel the other has shifted into a relaxed and open state.

- I often pick up that it's over or hear *It's done.*

- This depends. I often just feel it is time to end the session knowing that the person will benefit from coming back for more sessions. There is a sense to come to closure even though the field may not feel as rebalanced as it could be. Then comes the message, "It is better to underdo than overdo."

- For the most part I just know—I can tell by the way my being feels. It is another form of stillness. Almost what I would call a peace and a completion in this moment.

- This is an area where I need work. I always want to know the areas are all balanced, with no murky prana lurking in the healee's field. Sometimes it's obvious because the healing partner sighs or moves from side to side or come out of the "TT trance." Sometimes the person is kind enough to have his whole field come into balance and hold. Of course, if someone is immediately post-op, has been in terrible pain for a long time, or is very ill, we might temporarily get to this point or almost to it but it may not hold. I reassess and sometimes ask the healee what he is noticing. Often he is feeling quite good, despite my noticing some areas for further work. When I find myself going over the same areas the same way, that is often a time to stop. Sometimes I'll find my mind drifting, and centering produces a sense of needing to attend to something. Sometimes I start to smile.

- She looked very peaceful and needed very gentle short, light energy, and I just knew it was enough—any more would maybe have had an adverse effect.

- I always ask if the client feels anything else needs work. Sometimes I'm done at that point; other times, there is more. The client may ask for another area or two for additional attention. My healees are mostly oncology patients and I always feel as if I could work on them forever. I usually draw to a close when I feel with my hands that there is no more drawing of energy from them, or as with the adrenals, I feel intuitively that the area has received enough energy to rebalance itself.

⚘ I was unclear whether the session was finished on the treatment table. We ended it at my direction when his field was full and flowing into his feet, and resumed our conversation. I listened to him with my heart more open than previously and it occurred to me that possibly he had taken on illness in multiple organ systems as a metaphor for his life's work, experiencing disconnection, fighting against himself and illness in his body. I asked him if he has taken on other people's pain. "Oh yes," he said. "My heart is very big and I take on other people's troubles." I spoke aloud from my heart, advising, "Please let it run through you into the ground. Love your body." "All of it, even the pain?" he asked. "Yes. All of it. Fighting it is not the answer. Find compassion for your *self* and stop blaming yourself for your illnesses." He said as he left that no doctor had ever approached him beneath his symptoms. "They have always given me more pills." (I'd encouraged him to stop the excessive vitamin C, get out in sunshine, find a way to celebrate his birthday, and do activities he enjoys.)

⚘ There is a peace and fullness. The healing partner may appear more relaxed, but the sense of peace is within me. I close my eyes and there most likely will be a golden light in my mind's eye. As I rest my hands on the feet of the healing partner there is an easy and peaceful sensation in my hands. As I release the feet I feel a softness and/or puffiness—a feeling of big white clouds—in the area around the healing partner.

⚘ I noticed I came to alert presence in the room. My shift to done seemed to occur suddenly. Looking back, I could see it had occurred. She said, "It felt as if you moved something out of my chest. I feel lighter." She laughed at herself, the first laughter I'd heard in this session.

Deepening Sensitivity

It has been found that the longer the healer and the healee interact during the TT session (within the twenty- to thirty-minute guideline), the more deeply they are able to penetrate each other's subtle fields; they become more sensitive to one another. Interestingly, this is so whether they are doing hands-on TT close to one another, or TT at a distance. To a significant extent, space and time as we know them do not seem to be particularly critical to the healing interaction. In addition, the energy that is involved in healing continues to integrate, sometimes even accelerating the healing process after the formal session. A period of rest or sleep after a TT session seems to reinforce this continued ordered healing process for the recipient.

The increasing ease of subtle-field penetration, noted above, seems to deepen the therapist's conscious empathic understanding of the healing partner, whereas the partner's ability to sense the therapist's fields may or may not be conscious; at best he may feel more of a haze of confidence in the therapist's ability to help or to heal. Regardless of the depth of his awareness, however, change has occurred in both cases, which can be attested to in subsequent sessions as a significant increase in sensitivity, as experienced by the therapist and possibly by the partner. This increase in sensitivity, particularly in the therapist, should be fostered, but extra care should be taken to safeguard her continued health (staying alert to any symptoms of fatigue or anxiety in herself) at this time because of the vulnerability it engenders. For this reason, at the end of a TT session the therapist should give herself a period of quiet rest or do a simple meditation of ten to twenty minutes before she sees her next client or begins other acts of daily living.

Recall Phase

Therapists were asked: Do you have dreams, reveries, or any manner of interaction at a distance with your healing partner after the TT session? Which, and how often?

Dreams and Reveries

    ✎ I get periodic messages or insights (sometimes out of nowhere or just before falling asleep or getting up in the morning). I connect with the healing partner at a distance to send peace and love and help to maintain the field until next session. Sometimes I dream and get a message to focus on a certain area. I still feel and see the healing partner's presence and connection after the person leaves—and sometimes with people who have transitioned.

- I often had dreams, visions of my hospice patients after they had died. All told me they were okay. In one dream I had the feeling of being the person who had died, what his body felt like, feeling the discomfort. I might get a clue or insight after a session about why the patient is experiencing/manifesting what he is in the physical or mental world.

- I have dreams of people I heal at a distance, as if they are telling me how they are feeling, a visit.

- I have dreams of this person I have treated. The dreams are clear and we are together. Often when I have these dreams I call or write to her.

- If I've done a distance TT session just before going to sleep, I often wake in the night and find that I'm still giving them a session. I continue the session in my mind's eye and then fall asleep again. Other than that, I don't connect with them. I find this odd, since I do have a deep connection when I am working with them. I do sometimes get a nudge to give someone a TT session. I always try to follow up on these hunches and get feedback. Usually there is a good reason for having done the TT.

- I know that my dream space is profound—really wonderful—and I always look forward to what will be revealed. I trust deeply in my dreams. They are real states of consciousness that even after fifty-odd years I am still only glimpsing. I pay attention.

- I often think of people with whom I've had a TT connection even though I know nothing else about them personally. I feel like we are connected on some subtle level forever.

- I do follow-up (20–40 percent of the time) with a distant connection that may be as simple as a reassuring meeting of the minds that my healing partner's life is on an improving track, or an actual distance TT session if that feels necessary.

◢ Gentle reflections of recall are pretty amazing. I realize that there are moments when I bring healing partners into my awareness; there are other times that they appear.

Recall Information for the Therapist

◢ I think of healees occasionally, sometimes using distance healing to connect to someone's Inner Self, or send a stream of healing compassionate thoughts as a bridge from my heart to his.

◢ My focus was on the healing partner finding work that would meet his needs, and a vision of him whole and healthy. I felt slight pressure in my heart chakra during focused sending.

◢ I think of my healing partner in different ways, sending peace and presence of the Holy Spirit, energies of support.

◢ Sometimes I dream about a session and get a message to focus on a certain area in the next session. Most often messages will come to me out of the blue—*So-and-so needs more of something.* This helps with the next session. I am often still working with someone after he's left. I still see and feel his presence and connection. Messages can also come to mind while I am driving or doing something like laundry or resting.

◢ Able to shift consciousness during recall of TT, atemporal and nonspatial. It seems that TT memories are accessible by having or recalling actual, similar, or parallel experiences.

◢ Healing partners are in my thoughts more often; I think of them in wholeness, send energy.

◢ After treating, I have an energetic template of the healee. I find myself able to revisit that session and bring back the experiences of the moment. I find that I become aware of situations that occurred to the healing partner after having treated him. For instance, one morning while getting ready for work I smelled smoke. I looked all around the house. There was no smoke, but I could not stop smelling smoke. When I got to work that morning, I found out that an employee whom I had treated that week had had a house fire. This is what I mean by the energetic template or connectedness.

Sometimes dreams of the healing partner come in vivid color. The dreams may guide me to something more that needs to be done, so I occasionally offer distance TT, visualize him and see a session happening. Sometimes more than dreams, I'll have a sight or feeling in my Inner Self that cues me to another thing that could be done for a healee. I see in my mind's eye a session for that person. I usually close my eyes and see him; this happens as I am coming from the session, or a day later.

I was enormously relieved after the TT session, as we had returned from the crisis of the allergic reaction to the bee and adrenaline that masked her other symptoms. She was emotionally undone, which opened her to the physical issues (chronic bronchitis, excess smoking, and so on), that compounded her allergic symptoms, serious otitis leading to dizziness and falling, increasing her anxiety). Thank you, Inner Self, I couldn't sort that all out rationally. Also, this day I would have been exhausted without the benefit of TT on me.

During the treatment at our practicum session, one of the healers "saw" a golden beam of light. When the healee Z also "saw" the golden beam she decided to bring it in, as instructed, into her throat and heart. I saw the color of her field change suddenly from blue to a diffuse gold. Others felt a whoosh. Z "felt" the light go through her whole body. She felt her headache begin to dissipate and the cramped muscles in her back release. Those of us observing and holding the space could feel the energy smooth out and flow evenly into her legs. Z called me the next day to thank me for inviting her to the TT group and for "hanging in there with her" all these months. She didn't understand what had happened but she was very grateful and felt as if she had let go of important old stuff. She had returned home, slept well after the healing. Next morning her headache, which had been present for three months prior to the TT session, returned a little. She was able, with effort, to find the golden light and it dissipated. Laughingly she said it had been much easier to find with six of us [the members of the TT practicum group] helping in the treatment.

Conclusions

Below is a compilation of the major conclusions of this study. A few of the findings were admittedly serendipitous, but all are within the context of what is the essential purpose of this initial exploratory study: an inquiry into the idea of the experiential knowledge of healing, as seen from the perspective of the Therapeutic Touch therapist. It is hoped that this probe will point the way for others who will follow what, even now, can be perceived as a fertile field for further study in-depth.

Therapeutic Touch is an individual healing encounter that includes the following elements:

1. It takes into account the healing partner's needs as well as the Therapeutic Touch therapist's goals, experience, learning habits, culture, personal rituals, and beliefs.
2. A significant growth of the therapist's conscious self-awareness occurs during the TT process, along with deep realizations of the validity of the therapist's personal relationship to her Inner Self.
3. Over time there is a mentoring/overshadowing of the therapist by her Inner Self as mentor. This is of particular importance for the future consciousness of the TT process.
4. Stillness is a distinctive motif and accompaniment of the TT process. The profound stillness that occurs at the onset of the TT healing session and continues throughout that period is significantly correlated with the therapist's experience of the presence of the Inner Self.
5. Very often healing experience is bound by the limitations of verbal expression, but whatever metaphor the therapist uses, it becomes a figurative representation of her reality of the moment.
6. There is a realization that during the TT approach, a psychic bridge may be formed between the therapist and the healing partner.
7. The continued practice of Therapeutic Touch lends pattern and organization to the therapist's higher cognitive states and potentiates the functionality of abilities such as clairvoyance, mind-to-mind communication, intuition, and clarity.
8. The mature therapist may clearly visualize the problems of the heal-

ing partner during the TT search in healing at-a-distance, as well as during on-site healing. This vivid visualization seems to be coupled with intuition.

9. During the recall phase the therapist may discern deeper understanding of the healee's issues.

10. The experience of Therapeutic Touch is understood at the transpersonal level, for both the therapist and the healing partner.

An interesting second order finding is that space and time do not seem to have the same control over outcomes of the healing session as they do over other human behaviors. This lends itself to future consciousness of the Therapeutic Touch process.

7

"Looking Over My Shoulder"
Case Studies

The following studies detail experiences of trained therapists with three or more years of experience who agreed to participate in research into the process of Therapeutic Touch in-person healing.

Case 1

Stillness and Peace While Living with Cancer

Cancer presents challenges that are physical, emotional, and spiritual.

Approach

We walk together into the treatment room. It is comfortably dark with the light of the sunset pouring in through large windows. We see the skyline in the distance, the shadows illuminating the outline of what she and I call "city life." We smile, sit down face to face, and talk just a bit. I feel the quiet permeating the space . . . I am present to her and the sound of her voice. She shares a bit of her story with me and as she talks tears bubble up amid a smile of courage. Within my being I am still, profoundly so, and the feeling that encompasses me is what I will call a shared connection in this space . . . we are one, we are two . . . we are self in connection to other. My sense is that sense of standing in the sunlight under a blue sky, a feeling state of stillness with ears . . . and heart . . . and being open to discovery.

Outreach

As we walk together we hold hands. It seems to be a way of connection that she responds to, and as we talk we continue to hold hands. As I begin the treatment I place my hands on her shoulders.

Search

I am open to the ways that cues appear, the ways that information is revealed to me. Overall I sense a deep fatigue that transcends the physical challenges of living with cancer. It is this, yet more—a void, an emptiness, an emptiness emanating from her heart. I believe that she is . . . as strange as it sounds now and felt at the moment . . . struggling to find the will to go forward—not just with treatment but to *go forward in her life.*

How do I know? I can see it in my mind's eye. As I continue I actually feel the emptiness . . . yes, I am centered . . . yes, of course I check that out . . . yes.

Rebalance

I begin with gentle smooth movements crown toward foot, with the intention to relax and be—be as open as comfortable—and so it is, back and front . . . interspersed with a "moment" (not linear) of holding my hand gently over her heart and actually sensing the rhythm manifest there. The stillness becomes deeper . . . it is a comfortable and profound stillness and we just are . . . I am holding her shoulders and seeing us together in the out-of-doors. And I know it is time so I begin more brisk movements with the intention of energizing, almost strengthening.

I am suddenly aware from this deeper place of her struggle of letting go and I send thoughts of peace—a beautiful blue peace—to her heart . . . no expectations . . . just peace. I am clear that if/when she can let go, her fatigue will lessen. I am clear that this is a process of her own time and I know that in this moment I am here to support her through gentle, peaceful intention, smoothing the flow, inviting her to feel rooted. I use my hands, not slow but not brisk, crown to foot—with the intention of order . . . flow . . . rhythm . . . peace.

I touch her feet for grounding, and as we end our treatment she rests for ten minutes. I notice tears. I sit quietly.

What chakra do I use? I would say my crown and my heart direct my hands; my brow is vibrant in this moment, offering me some clarity of the myriad of cues, and I am also clear that my root chakra is illuminating a need for strong foundations.

My posture is flexible, relaxed.

Done

For the most part I just know, I can tell by the way my being feels. It is another form of stillness . . . almost what I would call a peace and a completion in this moment.

Recall

I have continued treating her at a distance. At first we scheduled every week; we had discussed this but soon realized that trying to set a day and time would be cumbersome so we decided together that I would share TT with her every week *and* that if she felt so inclined she would sit quietly and bring me to her mind.

My distance treatments include my bringing myself to her and sharing TT. Gentle reflections of recall . . . an interesting word . . . are pretty amazing. I realize that there are moments when I bring patients into my awareness, there are other times that they appear. I also know that my dream space is profound—really wonderful—and I always look forward to what will be revealed. I trust deeply in my dreams . . . they are real, states of consciousness that even after fifty odd years I am still only glimpsing. I pay attention.

Case 2
Chronic Pain and Deep Grief

Illness and medication inconsistency presented challenges to both the therapist and the person seeking healing.

Approach

I met C in my office. I noticed how tired and sad she seemed from the first moment she entered. I asked her how her life had been going these past weeks since I'd seen her last. I felt my hands begin to feel warm, as if they were ready to do TT work, so I asked "inside" if I should offer TT and got a large, silent *Yes*. I did not know if C would like TT but she immediately agreed to receive it and walked over to sit on the exam table. The warmth in my hands intensified as I walked across the room to begin.

Outreach

I held my hands over her adrenal glands and in contact with her low back to give her support. (I was conscious of her huge grief—both of her good friends have died this past year, leaving her with little female support. Her family is all involved in a huge family business, which is the source of much of her and her husband's stress.) I moved my hands through her field and felt a quiver in my right palm. (She has multiple sclerosis and I felt this odd electric quiver once before with another MS patient.) I moved my hands next to her body and noticed how "closed in" her field was. I held one hand on one side of her chest and the other hand on the other side. Her field began to fill in and I could tell that her field became more even.

Search

I start with hands heavy, reassuring on her physical shoulders. I move to physically support her at the adrenals and then low back. I caress her field around the torso with heart through my hands and feel her field fill. I move to her feet and physically draw my hands down her legs. I assess the flow near her ankles with my hands and look up at her heart with "soft eyes" and sixth (ajna) chakra. I see the churning there and watch the lovely slow swirls of the grey-white energy flows in her torso and heart. I notice a soft pink-blue in her field as we are finishing. Mentally I know she has chronic pain and physical issues, but I seem to be working primarily with her emotional field today.

Rebalance

I moved my hands downward along her legs and touched her skin to invite the field to move out of her chest and torso. I held my hands on her feet. I softly closed my eyes and saw lots of light around her torso and several splotches of dark near her heart. I offered energy from the universal field through C's field as I moved my hands across her chest front and back to move out whatever needed to flow out of her. I assessed and "used" my heart chakra as much as possible as well as my sixth chakra—inner eye. I intended love and support to her. I noted that her field had become more even and full adjacent to her feet. This helped me know she was rebalanced. She stayed deep in reverie even after I had completed and began to chart.

Done

I noticed my eyes had opened and that I had returned to a state of alertness and in-the-room consciousness. I completed TT with my hands and stepped away to chart from a nearby chair. She remained in deep reverie. Eventually I gently offered her a glass of water. I commended her on how well her body had responded to our work.

Recall

She has struggled with a tendency to addiction and excessive use of her antianxiety medications, and recently had to change pharmacies. She is striving to get well but has been challenging for me at times. Her memory loss and neediness coupled with impulsively discontinuing her meds—and subsequent withdrawal symptoms—have sometimes proved heavy for me. Our TT session today healed much of that stress for me. I felt genuine love for her and was delighted to "feel" her responding under my hands.

Case 3

Sensing Anxiety during a Class Demonstration

This TT therapist and teacher offers a demonstration treatment given to a group attending their first class in Therapeutic Touch. Observing treatments is one of our traditional teaching strategies.

Approach

We are a class of twenty-five. B volunteers to be the guinea pig and receive a treatment as a demonstration to the group. She comes to the chair; I invite the twenty-four observing students to help both B and me by holding the space, being present and silent. B and I talk for a moment and I assure her that she will be safe and that although we are on center stage, it is still not at all about anything other than she and I together within the TT space. I realize that I have been here many times and have learned so very much about this part of the Foundations TT course that I teach. I know that much has been trial by fire—really—and I know that within the TT we share that it will be safe and clear and that we will connect. I stand a moment and breathe deeply. When I sense that beautiful stillness, I know that I am ready and we begin.

Outreach

When we talk I am kneeling in front of B; I am holding her hands as we talk. I then proceed as described earlier.

Search

I gently move my hands as a demonstration for these new TTers. Moving head to toe, I follow the process as we teach and learn it.

I sense that the flow of energy in the arms has a distinct left/right difference. I also immediately pick up what I would describe as anxiety. I notice what I would call prickly, hyperdynamic flow all over—I really sense that she is not in this moment grounded. My sense is that in her life she is moving from one thing to the next, yet not necessarily finishing any one of them. Seems a lot to notice from this "pass over" but I take a deep breath, check in with myself, and I know these cues are accurate.

Rebalance

I gently move my hands from her head toward her toes. I move to the unruffling phase and my intention is for relaxation. I am teaching a class . . . I am clear and mindful of demonstrating the movements for new students.

I stand at her back with my hands on her shoulders and envision the bright sun, and then send that feeling of calm aliveness. I move my hands from her shoulder to her hand with the intention of evening the flow.

I check in . . . and then I do an initial grounding . . . seeing her feet snuggled into the earth. I continue to move my hands crown toward foot with the intention of rhythm . . . peace . . . actually a sense of comfortable order. I am seeing and integrating a blue-green color, light tone . . . almost a breezy movement.

Her head is resting forward. She has closed her eyes during the treatment and her breathing is slow. I am aware that we are finished in this moment . . . the environment is more alive to me now. I think it is that I am shifting in my awareness of it somehow . . . the lights, sounds, presence of others. She rests for five minutes as I sit quietly.

What chakras do I use? I would say my crown and my heart direct my hands—my brow offers me glimpses of clarity. And my posture? Responsive yet ready, knowing this is a class.

Done

In this particular situation, all eyes upon us, I am intentional in keeping the treatment short and light. I am not sure "light" is the right word, but I know what I mean. Over the years of teaching I have learned—and this has been through personal exploration as well as talking with my teachers—that in the class I must be mindful of the students' potential vulnerability. There is a wide variety of folks in attendance and a myriad of possible responses.

Recall

This is a recent TT interaction and twice I have felt the presence of B and sent her smoothing thoughts. These thoughts have been expressed as color and the color is a rosy pink imbued with deep blue . . . not a color I thought up but one that came during our TT session and when she came into my awareness.

Case 4

TT at a Distance on an Injured Ankle

This session provides a striking example of vivid visualization.

Approach

I had received an e-mail from a fellow TTer asking for distance TT on her ankle, as she had just fallen down the steps to her basement, and it was swelling and painful. I immediately sat on my chair and moved into Deep Dee, bringing my colleague L to the forefront of my consciousness. Suddenly I was able to see myself in her house, approaching her as she was sitting on a large, soft armchair with her feet up on an ottoman. She appeared to be a bit "shocky," and I saw myself go to her and put my hand on her shoulder, instructing her to open her mouth and lift her tongue so I could administer a few drops of Rescue Remedy [a Bach Flower remedy]. I have done many, many distance TT sessions and this was the most clear, vivid experience of being with the healee I have ever had.

Outreach

As I was sitting in my chair, watching myself at L's house, my hands were moving in both realities, if that makes any sense. I don't have any specific recollection of my hand chakras, but generally they are at full alert.

Search

I watched myself then do a gentle clearing, unruffling, of her field. Moving down to her ankle fairly quickly, I was aware of my third eye's vibration in my Deep Dee consciousness. The ankle was swollen and beginning to discolor, and was shooting off lots of heat and electrical charges. Momentarily, I was able to feel her pain and her fear (in my solar plexus).

Rebalance

At that point I visualized L's ankle in an unswollen and healthy state, and asked her to do the same. My hands moved down and away in fairly quick sweeping motions. I brought "blue" in and around her field, especially around her ankle.

Done

When she relaxed and was breathing deeply and steadily, and the ankle energy was flowing more smoothly, I ended the treatment, reminding her to ice her ankle and take it easy. My consciousness then returned to the chair in my house and I opened my eyes. I have no idea how long I had been working, only that I felt as if I had come back from a very deep place. I did not think about L or her ankle again until two weeks afterward, when our TT group had its monthly practicum.

Two Weeks Later

While people were chatting, L asked me if I had done distance TT on her ankle, as she said she so clearly felt me there. She said her ankle had made remarkable improvement and was much less swollen and painful within a few hours. As she was telling this I recalled the session in my mind's eye, but thought she had injured her ankle before our last practicum, and that I had been physically present to treat her. In fact, I thought she was mistaken in her memory, and I began to correct her by saying, "No, we were actually here right after it happened." She tilted her head a bit, giving me a confused look, and I suddenly realized that I was mistaken. It *had* been a distance TT treatment. So I shared with the group how the experience was so vivid and clear that, even in my memory, I had been physically there doing the treatment.

Case 5, Part I
A Barking Dog Becomes an Ally

This was the first of two sessions in successive days. An account of the second session follows in Case 5, Part II.

Approach

I felt anxious as I drove up to F's house. I wondered if I would be able to help her. When she called me to schedule a TT session at her home,

I knew she was in acute distress; usually she is willing to see me at my office. She has suffered with depression and disabling anxiety for some time, but told me that this was much more intense than usual. As I walked into her backyard, her anxious terrier barked and pulled at his leash. He did not want me there. I attempted to center myself with limited success. F invited me into her bedroom to do TT. I noticed on the way through her kitchen that the sink was full of unwashed dishes. F lay down on her big bed and I tried to find a comfortable way to do TT with her. I noticed she looked pale and exhausted.

Outreach

My hands began to feel a little warm (the air-conditioned room was cool). My hand chakras connected with her arm as I waited a long moment to connect with her energy and grounded myself. "Good," I said, as I felt her take a deep breath. Since she was lying on her bed, I had to reach to get to her. I began to physically feel the closely held field of her body as I passed my hands close to her body. There was virtually no flow in her legs, and this became my first intervention. I stroked her legs physically again and again in a downward motion to get some flow going. Her body responded quickly. From where I was at her feet, I looked with my inner eye and saw a swirling blue and black in her torso and upper chest.

Search

Sequence of information: Noticing my gestalt in her house (irritable, slightly uncomfortable, noisy dog barking outside, objecting to my presence). Connecting with my hands and feel/know she is relaxing under their weight. I center more deeply as I am touching her. I move my hand chakras to discern her field and find it very close and thin. No flow in her legs. As we work, my hands warm more and I feel her field flow in response. It is "thicker" and readily present in her legs, where my hand is touching, near her feet. I use my third eye to visualize, and see swirling colors in her torso. I intentionally direct energy with my hands near her chest and abdomen. I feel the flow of her field down her legs with my hands adjacent to her legs.

I revisualize her field and "think blue," and then see a deep blue around her throat and chest. Surprised at its intensity, mentally I compare it to the very deep blue I have seen (while doing TT) around the throat of a dying person and decide that this is a lighter hue. There is a pale turquoise blue around the rest of her torso. I connect deeply with my hands "on" her adrenals and feel unsettled and a bit sick as the energy pulls me deeply, deeply and then grounds more fully. I feel physical compassion for her and wonder if this is a tiny bit of the discomfort and malaise that she feels regularly. I feel relief as I take a deep breath and know/"hear" that I am to move to another phase of the treatment.

Rebalance

Once the flow is going in her legs, I move my hands to her adrenals and hold them against her body. She says, "That's where most of my back pain has been." I move to clear her torso, and move my hands downward so the flow will go down her legs. Looking back up to the previous site of swirling blue and black, I "think blue" and in a few moments see a lovely deep blue color appear, especially around her neck and upper chest. I put my hands again on her adrenals and feel myself go deeper. I ground more, as the energy is very strong and almost unsettling as I connect deeply with her. I understand in my body how she can feel so sick from whatever this is. I feel intense compassion for her.

Bent over in the odd position to reach her adrenals I am nearly off balance, but deliberately grounded through my feet. It is a relief to feel finished for the moment with that area. Reassessing her flow, I find it fuller and smoother than it was earlier. She appears to be deeply relaxed. I am also aware of her barking dog in the distance. (He is a terrier, quite hyper and very connected to my patient. He knows I am a stranger in the house, and he is unhappily outside.) Sometimes he is quiet while we work. I wonder if he is tuning into her more relaxed state. Certainly the barking was barely noticeable compared to the major distraction it seemed to be when we first started.

Done

I palpated her field and found it smooth, even, and full. I noted her calm deep breathing and improved color in her face. I noticed that my attention was in wrap-up mode, checking for any last details I might have missed. I was "back" in the room, aware of the dog barking, of the color of the walls and bedspread. My mind was no longer within her field. I stood back, prayed/invited any last instructions from Inner Self, with my hand chakras a bit farther from her body than they had been. Complete.

Case 5, Part II
Day Two with an Injured Client and Her Dog

This was the second of two sessions in successive days, the first of which is detailed above.

Approach

F calmly welcomed me into her home. I began to ground and center as soon as I entered the house. Today the dog was also inside the house and was welcomed into the bedroom where we worked. The atmosphere in the house was more comfortable, less irritable and dusty than the day before. I could imagine being comfortable here. The dog lay quietly on the floor at the entrance to the bedroom and came up onto the bed uncertainly when invited. He gently licked her hand and lay with his nose against her leg and his paw on her flank. During the session he lay entirely quiet, "helping." I let my hands rest on her arms for a long moment as I centered more deeply. She breathed deeply. Her field was fuller than yesterday.

Outreach

I move toward F and rest my hands on her arm. My hands palpate the continued thickness and note the quality of her field. I feel the unevenness of her field around her chest, but I notice it has held and is fuller than yesterday around her torso, and is now flowing well in her legs. I work with the thin field adjacent to her legs.

Search

My hand chakras palpate her field and discover that although there is fullness around her torso, her legs do not have much fullness in their field. From my station at her feet, I "look" with inner eye and see swirling blue and black across her chest, but less pronounced than yesterday. I clear the field and put my hands on her adrenals. There is a good flow, but not the unsettling sick pull, as was the case yesterday. Using my hand chakras I feel an extra fullness around her chest and work to clear the area again. I stroke downward on her legs. Looking "up" toward her torso I "see" strands of green emerging from a brownish background, as if tendrils are forming, growing. I see flowing water as I stand and hold my hands over her chest. It does not flow in interrupted waterfalls like yesterday, but rather it is like a connected stream (flowing) into a larger lake.

I feel the even fullness of the field at her feet and welcome "down" anything that needs to come down. I see golden light around her chest and upper abdomen (third chakra). I invite Inner Self to let me know if there is anything more to do. I thank her angels for helping today. More fully aware and in the room, I notice the quiet dog resting comfortably and holding his position gently touching her.

Rebalance

Her field responded quickly to my presence and hand movements encouraging flow down her legs. (I could detect the flow before she claimed to be able to feel flow in her hands.) I physically touched her flanks, holding my hands over her adrenal glands. I cleared especially her chest and abdomen. I saw with soft eyes the colors around her change to a pink-blue magenta color as I worked. From her feet I saw the change in her swirling blue and black to emerging green tendrils over her chest and later a bright golden yellow. I saw a flowing stream. At the end of the session I felt sad and nearly shed a tear.

Done

I found I was fully back in the room, noticing the color of the walls and bedspread, and the position of the dog. I "tucked in" the end of her field at her feet and gently smoothed the surface of her field at a distance of about two feet from her body. I noticed my sadness and thanked my Inner Self and F's angels for their assistance.

Recall

F called me the afternoon following this treatment. She had felt strong enough to go to her doctor's office briefly, which had been an improvement over the day before. She told me that surprising to her, she had suddenly wept deeply after I left her house, for a long time. She had not realized she was sad, and "had nothing to weep about." I told her how delighted I was that she was allowing these (blocked) emotions to come forth. She admitted that she has been "holding on by a thread" for a very long time. She said that it has been a relief to finally let go and let in the nurturing "love" she felt during the session. We agreed to meet for another session soon.

Case 6

Calming a Chatty Injured Friend

A therapist experiences a deepening trust in the TT process.

Approach

My initial experience in approaching the healing partner was difficult. She was a friend who kept talking, and had just injured her knee; it was locked.

Outreach

My hand chakras were "on" and when they are in that phase, I sense them as little bowls.

Search

My hands picked up the info as "heat/warmth sensors." The involved chakras were hand and heart. The sequence was one of moving my hands from her head, downward through her field. Again she was very chatty, finally stopped, and I picked up that her injured knee was drawing energy; she was very depleted.

Rebalance

Sent energy to her knee by placing one hand behind the knee and moving hand in front, downward.

The healee was lying down, so I placed one hand under her at times, and to do so, as I'm tall, I put myself into a sort of L-shaped yoga position to protect my lower back, sticking my butt out and anchoring my feet and legs.

Chakras used: heart/hand and I imagine my crown is activated by the love I project. I know that my consciousness shifts once I begin picking up changes, the changes I've been instrumental in helping to take place. It's as though this is my evidence that the energy treatment is doing something. I'm still relatively new at this, though I've been doing TT for four years. Really new is how I have been feeling this year. The rebalancing experience that means the most for me is usually when I realize that the congestion has been directed down and out, and is out of the healee's field. I'm continually amazed at this.

Done

I know I'm done when nothing seems to be changing; I understand that a session should not go over twenty minutes at the most.

Recall

I enjoy treating friends and acquaintances because it's usually from these people that I get feedback. Maybe not right then, but a phone call later saying something like, "I went downstairs and could use both legs!" or, "My hip pain is gone; I could sleep all night and didn't even wake up." Honestly, this TT journey, for me, has been one of complete trust. Trust that something is really happening. It's very intriguing to me.

Case 7
The "Sound" of an Injured Field

Centering deeply in the impersonal space is essential when working with friends and loved ones.

Centering/Approach

The approach with H was our moving from chatting at the dining room table to getting her settled on a twin bed in a spare bedroom. H had fallen seven months ago and fractured bones in her lower leg, requiring surgery with pins and plates to put her together. About four months ago it was determined that some of the metal in her legs had cracked, requiring another surgery. Then just this past week H heard a crack in her left leg, the sound of metal cracking yet again. At the ER the following day the lower leg was splinted and temporarily cast. Today is Saturday; on Monday she will go to her regular surgeon's office but will have to see the assistant. This is a friend of whom I am very fond. This made the centering critical, to keep myself in the impersonal space, setting aside any of my personal feelings.

Outreach

After walking with her knee scooter to the bedroom, H got herself settled on the bed. We determined that a single pillow under her head was enough support. I did not notice any specific chakras getting involved. My focus was on the reality of H and myself as fields. I actually sense us as fields, sort of like clouds of gentle mist. Now as I recall the session, I do feel that without being consciously aware of it at the time, my heart chakra was doing the listening to H's field.

Search/Assessment

My palms moved through H's field from head to toe. I did a search through the left side of her body (she was supine) and then the right side. I also did a search with my mind through the back body, where I sensed the energy of fatigue. There was a disconnection of flow through her right arm. And on the whole right side the field seemed sorrowful—with even a "sound" of moaning. Of course, the right side has had to work harder since this new injury to the left leg.

Rebalance

Being aware of energy moving through the entire body and field, I first did a general clearing and felt a buoyancy begin to come into the field. Dee often talks about "clear light," and this was one of the feelings that came in as the quality of energy I was directing through her field. When I was bringing my hands through the field on the right side, I was guided to direct the qualities of "peace, wholeness, order," the words I said silently while moving my hands.

I took one of my hands at her back—one side at a time—and invited blue through the field from the back, sweeping my other hand through the field at the front, in a head-to-toe direction. I directed blue through the left leg for pain reduction (she is on painkillers) and then green for the healing of the cells of the bones. A hand at the back of the neck directed a gentle blue, as the other hand cleared at the front.

Done

The reassessment indicated some more generalized, balanced flow throughout; and on the right side, I got an image of the field of that whole side being "knitted" together. "Done" came to me when a thought of my own life dropped into my consciousness.

Recall

We have continued to be in touch pretty much daily as she networks to find an orthopedic ankle and foot surgeon. When she comes to mind, I can easily get the feeling of energetic flow through her body and spirit. She continues to embody the positive attitude she has had since the accident.

Case 8
Hospice Patient Awakens Unexpectedly

Staying centered helped to keep the therapist attuned in working with a formerly unresponsive healing partner.

Approach

This is my first visit to this young woman on hospice who has been slowly declining over many years with muscular atrophy. She was totally unresponsive, as had been reported to me. She was lying motionless and lifeless covered with blankets—face partially covered, eyes tightly shut, expressionless.

Outreach

I felt no connection to her Inner Self, but I centered and connected to my own Inner Self and was guided not to go near her head. I placed my hand chakras about ten inches above her body near the throat and very slowly and lightly moved my hands down to her feet one time.

Search

I maintain a sustained centered state, which keeps me connected to my Inner Self. I very clearly follow the guidance of my inner voice—and the more centered I am, the more I feel I am connected to my healing partner's Inner Self, the more information I receive on what to do. And I am reassessing continually as I am treating—I think sometimes it is my right hand treating and my left hand assessing or getting information and I just follow along with an effortless effort and know that I am not *doing* it but staying in the flow of the universal energy field. The more deeply I am centered, the deeper the connection is with my healing partner.

Rebalance

I am usually standing and walking around the bed or chair during assessment, usually ending at the feet. I often start with a light massage of the feet to help my healing partner to relax, while also observing and assessing the body. For this session I picked up information from her foot and my hand chakras (like hand-foot connection). I absolutely knew there was a shift in consciousness—she woke up! Her eyes opened! She was looking at me! I felt guided to start playing soft, joyful harp music and then to do hand-heart connection.* Her right hand was in a tight contracted grip (her left hand is paralyzed), so I slipped my finger

---

*Cathleen Fanslow, *Using the Power of Hope to Cope with Dying: The Four Stages of Hope* (Fresno, Calif.: Quill Driver Books, 2008), 104. (The hand-heart connection technique was developed "to help families and other direct caregivers maintain necessary contact and to help decrease the feelings of helplessness and pain.")

into her hand and felt a tremor, and then I felt her holding my finger. I sat next to her for several minutes. I asked her if she would like me to come back. She mouthed "Yes." When I said goodbye she mouthed "Bye." Seeing her wake up, I felt it was clear that she had become more balanced. I had been told she couldn't speak.

Done

She looked very peaceful and needed very gentle, short, light energy, and I just knew it was enough—any more would maybe have had an adverse effect.

Case 9

After Hip Replacement

A therapist feels through the layers of the field to restore balance.

Approach

I was comfortable with J. We had shared a dinner I cooked; I'd asked that she relax and allow me to do TT for her. She was post-surgery for a bilateral hip replacement.

Outreach

It took more than a moment to center. Our conversations had been deep during dinner and when we were in the positions—J on her bed and me kneeling beside her—my hands were anxious to begin. I took three more breaths and really allowed myself to center. Finally I allowed my hands to pass from head to toe and they were alive, willing, and ready to pick up any cues, any sensations. They were connected to my brain in a straight-line connection, and I got the message, "Don't forget her arms."

Search

There are layers of information. On the surface I think the sensations I feel relate to pain, circulation, physical functioning of J's body. There is something in the upper back, something cool around the feet, something huge in her head. As I work through these requests for shifts, another layer is exposed and here I think I am beginning to touch the emotions that underlie the physical expression. I work as before from head to toe but allow myself to enter a deeper connection with the cues and work from the front to address a disturbance on J's back. The emotional field seems less able to receive directly. Is there a sequence? I suppose the sequence is physical, emotional, and ethereal. The final round of TT is where I ask J's ancestors to continue to work with her, and my hands are moving more to encourage and support than shift any energy.

Rebalance

For J yesterday there was the sense of wondrous healing in the hips but a reluctance to allow energy to flow completely down her legs. Today I moved from the regular flowing movements of TT to holding her feet. Because she was in bed and I was beside her it was hard to hold her feet symmetrically, although at first I tried, so I worked one foot at a time. I was aware of a need to support the flow through J's feet and this I did by physically touching and encouraging movement . . . aliveness . . . awareness. My hand chakras were key, but I think my root chakra was also strongly aware of what was going one. Gently holding . . . barely moving . . . one foot at a time, working through J's foot chakras but also right down to her toes. I watched the energy shift and begin to flow. Satisfied, I covered her feet and went back to hands-off TT.

Done

On reassessing I found the initial cues were no longer there. There was lightness above J's head, the energy flowed smoothly down her back, there was no congestion or disturbance around her hips, and energy flowed both down her arms and legs. Her feet, which had been cool, were warm. I tucked J into bed, sensing the human bond was as critical to healing as the TT.

Recall

Perhaps it is too early to dream about J, but I awoke this morning aware that three others in my community needed TT—dealing with metastasized colon cancer, back pain, and a broken heart—and will meditate then send TT to them and out to the universe, where it will be directed to where it is needed.

Connecting Deeply with Healing Partner with Broken Neck

A therapist is able to move from surprise and concern to an Inner Self–to–Inner Self connection.

Approach

To give you the picture of my experience, I need to describe the situation I encountered. K had just sustained a broken neck, having fractured two cervical vertebrae while jumping on a trampoline with his kids a few days prior. When I went to his home he was wearing a heavy plastic neck brace, walking around and lifting two small dogs to put outside, as well as the chair he would sit on while I did TT. My initial response was of surprise, as I did not expect him to be so active with a broken neck. I noted that I started to assess his energy field while he was moving around. I immediately sensed anxiety and anger. When he sat on the chair, I sensed/validated his behavior was one of denial and challenge and he was not accepting the severity of his injury.

Outreach

Hands are tingling. Sensing an erratic field. Anything else? Anxious to get to doing treatment with TT.

Search

I started with my third eye and crown, then the heart sensing and solar plexus kicked in trying to make sense of this man who was running around as if he did not have a broken neck. My heart sensed the physical and emotional pain. My third eye went deeper into sensing any communication from his field, mind-to-mind—Inner Self to Inner Self. Note: With this healing partner I felt a strong connection deep in my soul with his soul. All of my energy centers were connected to his; it was like our souls were old friends reconnecting. This has happened before, but rarely. In any sequence I generally start with the third eye, solar plexus, and crown chakra, and often the heart center. At times and dependent on the partner, different chakras may get involved.

Rebalance

I did a lot of smoothing of the shoulder area to help him to relax. He was tight and had a pattern of carrying everything on his shoulders. He was also very tight in the shoulder area as a protection of his recently fractured vertebrae. I acknowledged it and had him do some deep breathing while I smoothed his shoulders and cleared around the area of the pain in his neck.

How do you know when your state of consciousness shifts? My state of consciousness shifts right away when I am about to work with a healing partner. I center from the time I start to interact with him, from the time of our fields connecting, from our first greeting. I then experience another shift into a deeper consciousness when I begin to assess the field and then throughout the process. I cannot describe it as a different level of consciousness; I am in another state of being. My being and the healee's being are interconnected and communicating in subtle ways. With K, I felt a soul connection had been reunited. The communication in this case was easy and profound.

The rebalancing experience is dependent on what I sense in the assessment and connection with chakras and Inner Self to Inner Self. I felt K needed to have the pain in his neck and arm reduced before he could relax. I smoothed and cleared the areas. He had a bone chip in his neck, which caused severe pain and weakness in his left arm. I sent energy to the neck and throat area, then worked with the nerves to help rebalance and reduce pain in his arm by sending loving and peaceful energy to the neck area and down the arm through the fingers. It is like working in layers for me. For K, it was first the relaxation and partial pain relief. When the pain began to lessen, I was drawn to his heart area to send energy for him to rebalance and calm his heart center. He was very angry and fearful. I was drawn to direct calm, unconditional love through his heart area and whole being. The areas of pain and injury, his heart and throat, were all calling for attention. After this I was drawn to again concentrate on helping him relax by smoothing of shoulders, face, and neck areas—gentle smoothing with the intention again of sending rebalancing, relaxing, loving, and peaceful blue-violet energy.

Generally when I work my back is straight and I move up and down with my knees. The energy flows so much better through me that way. I am more open to accept messages from chakra to chakra. I use my chakras from the time I encounter my healee. I have always just taken this for granted as I realize I have done this since I was a small child. Upon initial encounter my third eye and solar plexus are at work assessing the energy, the healing partner's chakras for any connection. I am in tune both cognitively and energetically/intuitively from the beginning. By the time I begin the hands-on session, so to speak, I have already connected with the healing partner energetically and intuitively. I follow the guidance of my third eye, heart, and solar plexus throughout the session. I pick up messages both intuitively and through a voice in my ear or head. Sometime I get a picture of the problem in my mind's eye and watch as it is rebalanced.

Centeredness is the key. It is so easy to stay in this space, and it is what K needed to experience from me—heart-centered unconditional love and peace. Messages come to me from mind-to-mind connection; in other words, Inner Self to Inner Self. From this space I do the session. For this person I find that gentle smoothing of his shoulders in the field with some light touch relaxes him and opens him to accept the TT healing and rebalancing. I follow direction from Inner Self. Hands on, hands off works best with helping him to rebalance.

Done

I determined the session was complete when I noted his energy was balanced and flowing more freely. Even though there were areas of some imbalance, the field was not readily accepting any more energy and he needed to process the session and allow the energy to absorb and to process. He was visibly relaxed and relieved.

Recall

No dream, I get periodic messages or insights post session. For example, I'll be driving along and a message will come out of nowhere or when meditating just before falling asleep or getting up in morning. With K, the day after this session a message came as I was doing some house-cleaning that his spiritual being was in pain and to be sure to connect with this part of him on a deeper level next session.

Case 11

Sensing the Soft Heart in a Skeptical Patient

As the therapist stays present with a skeptical patient, we see again that even when the conscious mind holds resistance, the field of the person may be open to change.

Approach

I observed his posture, how L was walking and moving, where he was stiff, and how he was breathing in his body. Feeling into his fields, I noticed some accustomed patterns of behavior. It felt specifically about belief systems, some rigidity, what I interpret as his *true* beliefs. Overall the energy emitting from his fields had rigidity but also a soft heart—a caring person who holds himself and his beliefs with sternness and reluctance to let go or change.

Search

I am picking up information with my hand chakras, which I feel send the information into my whole system, and then I let the information, in a sense, run through my chakras. The search happens against my background of being centered and relaxed into the intelligence of my chakras and my Inner Self—the experience of my wholeness. Then I compare what I pick up from L to this background of centered Inner Self wholeness.

It seems that I am listening through my hands and my chakras—heart, crown, and brow almost simultaneously. My hands transmit the information to my heart and root chakras, then usually crown and brow. But at the same time my chakras are also picking up info. The crown chakra is very helpful to me for "order." Root chakra is important for my own grounding. Heart chakra is essential to simply connect with universal peace and my Inner Self. The brow chakra shows me pictures, and I also see some of the energy fields.

Once I get the info, then I let it sift through the intelligence of my chakras and the background living-energy of wholeness, order, and compassion, and wait and listen from my Inner Self and let it "talk" to me.

Rebalance

I relax purposefully in my body and my fields so that he will feel "relaxation in the air." I make sure he is physically comfortable. He has checked in with me verbally and now I quiet and set a standard of energy in the room, so to say, of time to quiet. I purposely connect with order from my crown chakra and compassion from my heart chakra.

In my body position I just relax; I have proper alignment in my physical structure in whatever position I assume. I use the heart, crown, brow, and root chakras, especially heart chakra for integration.

I know my consciousness shifts when I feel integrated, I don't feel worried about the outcome, I feel aligned with my Inner Self and the energy of wholeness, order, and compassion. I feel at ease.

The rebalancing experience that holds the most clarity takes place when I am working with his inflamed liver, feeling into the tissues, sending blue then as I continue to feel into the tissues, to understand them; under the inflammation is an energetic connection to his heart chakra. Aha! An insight that liver inflammation is related to how energy flows through his solar plexus chakra. (Later I realized it was his heart chakra involved, not his solar plexus.)

Of course in the rebalancing there is continued assessment. I find that now I take my time and try to clue into the order in which I should unravel the imbalance(s). And this order comes from my continued connection through my Inner Self to that universal healing energy comprised of order, wholeness, and compassion. I often find that I feel I am missing a piece of the picture, so I have learned to sit back into my heart chakra and listen again to the healing partner's field from that place of consciousness. I often remind myself of the "natural human potential for healing"—that potential. If I focus on the energy of potential, I am usually rewarded with an insight as to how to continue (even if the "continue" means to be finished, either because I have reached my limit or the partner has reached his).

Done

Things have moved more toward order, I can feel it in his fields; he is relaxed and there is a sense that this is all he and his fields are able to do right now. It's a sense of healthy saturation. It is interesting to see him softening not only in his body but also an opening in his mind. He is more receptive all of the time to TT, where before he pooh-poohed it.

Recall

It wasn't until two days afterward, actually during meditation, that I realized the aha I'd had was really about his heart chakra. At the time I remember I immediately associated the imbalance with his solar plexus chakra, as that chakra is very disrupted for him. This gives me insight into what to look for next time I see him.

Case 12

Connection with Oak Tree Assists Deepening Wholeness

After surgery relieved a physical blockage in the small intestine, TT provided healing on the level of the subtle energies.

Approach

M was obviously fed up with this ailment. She'd recently had surgery for a blocked small intestine and a portion of her small intestine had to be removed. She was having a hard time staying on the liquid diet and wanted to eat as she normally would, but each time she did she ended up back in the hospital with pain. Both frustration and tears were present as we greeted each other.

Outreach

My hand chakras were trying to get a feel for what is going on in her system, as well as what is going on with her mentally and emotionally. My hands were passing through her field, getting to know her field today. Today, I was also trying to "hear" more with my hands, letting them stay awhile in her field without the need to rebalance just yet . . . listening to hear more of the rhythms of her field. The rhythms feel confused to me today . . . lots of conflicting information coming in and now my hands are simply being with this energy and trying to sort it into some order or sense.

As I look back I realize that my hands were doing a few things: first, just feeling the field, getting to know the field, asking the field to reveal itself to me; second, gathering information that was being transmitted from my hand chakras to my heart, crown, root, and brow chakra; and third, opening the field a bit so that I could get that information.

Search

How am I picking up information? My hand chakras are transmitting some of the information to me, but also my own entire field is picking up information. I'm aware of my emotions feeling her emotions; my mind feeling her state of mind. I'm also aware of her patterns of stress and her nervous system. I don't understand it all yet, but I'm getting this information and also letting myself consciously and purposefully open to her and her information. I'm also aware of really grounding myself and breathing slowly and deeply to be quiet, to center in that place of inner quiet so that I can listen.

What chakras are kicking in? My crown, heart, hands, solar plexus, brow, and root chakras.

Is there a sequence? Can I describe it? I have been treating M on and off over the past few weeks. It seems so clear to me that part of her continuing difficulty is her resistance to having this condition. If I am to help her, I feel that I need to get underneath the symptoms and support her on a deeper level of how she engages, unconsciously or consciously, with the situations of everyday life, and help her to see more easily and clearly her patterns and to choose whether they are helpful to her or not. But these insights have to spring from within her, not from my telling her; that goes only so far.

So today I am very intentionally reaching into my Inner Self and connecting with wholeness and the universal life/healing energy. My heart chakra is the door for this. The sequence would be my centering into my own Inner Self/consciousness through my heart chakra, then using my hand chakras to move through her field; then the information is disseminated to my heart, crown, root, and brow chakras. I listen to the information I receive from each one of these. It feels like the info all floats by and through my centers of consciousness, and from the background of my Inner Self an understanding emerges of how to engage and proceed with her.

The information doesn't all come at once. There seems to be an initial gathering of information that gives me enough to have an overall picture as well as a starting place for the rebalancing. But as the treatment continues and the more the "surface" cues are rebalanced, I find that I am searching once again with my hand chakras in her field and from my Inner Self, asking *What else*? This is when I find the deeper imbalances of dysrhythmia within her chakra system, and especially how her nervous system's habit pattern of disrupting her digestion comes to light. Again, it is listening from my Inner Self (heart chakra) as my hands are passing through her field and that information is then transmitted through my chakra system, and I am listening from that living experience of natural order that I can connect to through my Inner Self.

Rebalance

How do I know when my state of consciousness shifts? When I think back on this, usually I have an insight as to how to continue with the treatment. There is a bit of creative chaos that happens as I am gathering information. It all seems to be spinning within my consciousness (the intelligence of my chakras and my connection to universal healing energy). As I sit with this, there seems to be a coming together of this information and then an insight as to how to continue. This usually feels right, a sense of *Okay . . . aha, yes, let's travel down this path.*

Do I use certain chakras? My hands and heart certainly seem to be the leader today, but also as I continued into the treatment and wanted to find out more about the underlying tension, I kept going to my crown chakra and peering, so to say, from there and listening. Then I had to relax back into that connection with natural order and wholeness and compassion to let the information run through that energy and listen again, as this seemed to then make sense within me as to how to proceed.

Do I hold my body in certain positions or postures? I just simply try to relax my body. It seems that when I withdraw to center into my deep center, I often find that my hands (or one hand) are at my heart center . . . I just realized that. It is very helpful for me to sink physically into my feet. I'm learning t'ai chi right now and I find that it is helping me to sink into my feet more easily and feel supported physically from this.

How do I assist my healing partner to shift into rebalance? First we talk for a few minutes and I acknowledge her frustration at this situation. Then we go upstairs and she lies on the bed. I ask about her comfort. Once she is physically comfortable, then I continue. For M today it was important to spend some time talking about her illness and her frustration and for her to feel heard, not answered so much as simply heard.

Then holding her feet and letting her settle down into her body was very helpful, encouraging her to breathe down her body and out her feet. I offered simple instructions as her irritation level was very high and it felt like too much direction would not be helpful. For myself, I consciously withdrew energetically for a few moments, aligned with my deep center, and relaxed into my body and my heart center. I used my field as a mirror for her field to feel relaxation, so I consciously relaxed—physically, mentally, and emotionally.

Toward the end of the treatment the physical pain had been reduced and superficial symptoms relieved to a degree but she had not deeply relaxed and I felt that deep healing, really shifting healing, had not taken place. I could feel that what would really help would be if she could deeply relax enough that I could reach her underneath her habit patterns of how she runs her nervous system. I might also be able to reach the disordered pattern in the way that the spleen chakra and her digestive system were not working together, how they were adversely affected by her anxiety. It also felt like her heart chakra was not fully present in the equation (I'm often finding this now with many people), the healthy integration of natural and whole flow was not present. This is the place I wanted to reach.

How to do this? I closed my eyes and went even deeper into my Inner Self. There is a big, beautiful oak tree in their yard that I could see from the window, so I connected with the tree and asked it to help me. I had to calm myself a lot and deeply relax into my heart chakra and connect with my Inner Self. When I had that experience of relaxation and deep quiet and connection to universal wisdom (that is how I experience the Inner Self), and I felt solid in that connection, I then expanded out/reached out from my Inner Self to her Inner Self with the intention of connecting with her innate wholeness. This seemed important to effect the change I was after to connect with her innate wholeness, her Inner Self wholeness. As I did this her energy started to change. She fell into a deep sleep and then I felt I had access to the underlying patterns of imbalance. I did not have to "do" anything except be present with this wholeness and engage my hands in this flow of energy that was present and help it to move around and through her different organs and chakras. But it was more that I was engaged in the dance at this deep core level and in a sense allowing and supporting her innate wholeness to do its job that it couldn't do on its own, as she would get in the way of it.

This felt like a healing moment—where the underlying pieces of the puzzle were aligned with her innate wholeness. Her field was the clearest I had ever felt it. Integration was happening. Unobstructed flow was happening. And I could reach it only through the Inner Self.

Done

How did I know that the TT treatment was complete? What else was there to do? We were definitely done. I stayed in her field until it felt that the reorganizing (I did not have to do anything except stay connected and present, and the healing energy did the work) was finished, and there was such a beautiful glow happening. She was deeply asleep, so we were done.

Recall

I have thought about this treatment often, remembering the connection with wholeness and what it felt like to reach that depth/stage and the resulting effortless rebalancing/healing—truly a healing moment—that happened. I'm very grateful for that experience.

Case 13

Phantom Limb Pain: Two Sessions

P had a traumatic above-knee amputation of his left leg twenty-eight years ago, and for the past eighteen years has had phantom pain in the amputated leg that no pain pills have been able to relieve. The therapist has been doing treatments twice a month for a year.

Approach

Week One: He was smiling and there was an acceptance in his field.

Week Two: Acceptance and waiting for me to begin TT.

Outreach

Week One: Moving from the head downward, assessing the differences in the field and the level of the differences from the physical body.

Week Two: Moving downward from his head to his feet, assessing for differences from one side to the other with my hand chakras. I concentrated on clearing the energies over his abdomen and left thigh stump during the assessment phase.

Search

Week One: I was picking up information from my hands, which then seemed to be integrating into my field and causing an intuitive thought (sixth chakra?) about the healing partner. My hand chakras sensed a field of energy about twelve inches beyond his stump. He mentioned that he could feel my touching his leg, a part of which is now gone. My intuitive thought during the treatment was that this was an emotional pain, a sense of holding on to the experience.

Week Two: After doing the initial assessment with my hand chakras, I went to his stump to assess the distance of the energies from the stump and found that the energies stopped at the physical stump. P felt this at the same time I noticed it in the field. Both of us were pleasantly surprised. I took a deep breath to re-center, and continued the treatment.

Rebalance

Week One: P is always in a reclining chair, so I am usually in a kneeling or leaning-over posture. I started to rebalance by moving to his head in an erect position. After the reassessment, I felt a shift to my heart chakra as I facilitated grounding at his shoulders and feet.

Week Two: I moved from kneeling at his left side to his shoulders, standing erect at the back of his recliner chair. I sent energy from my hand chakras and sent peace and comfort from my heart. I felt the shift in energy centers in the physical body but also within my own field— which is not as defined as physical touch but more like a knowing and sensation.

Done

Week One: He seems very relaxed and the field is nearly balanced.

Week Two: His field usually has some mild imbalances at reassessment but if I have been there for twenty to twenty-five minutes and he seems relaxed or is napping, I terminate the treatment and finish with the intention of grounding at his lower extremities.

Recall

Week One: I often ponder a way to explore my thoughts about the emotional aspects of his trauma. This is his first experience of energy work and he has gone from skeptical to accepting. I have taught him imaging several times, which he does not do.

Week Two: I have been thinking about him more often. He has lost a son and older brother within a couple of months. I send him peace and the presence of the Holy Spirit.

Case 14

Healing for Persistent Anxiety

In a relationship established over some years, trust in the therapist allows a healee to relax.

Approach

R and I have shared a relaxing morning . . . enjoying breakfast, chatting, sharing our dreams, both personal and professional—is there really a difference? We move to our beautiful space overlooking the gardens and the woods. As I move to begin sharing TT, I first look deeply at R, then gaze for a moment out the window. There is a profound stillness; I can feel it in every bit of my being and I can hear it—the music of silence.

Outreach

I place my hands on her shoulders as we, together, take a few breaths and look out the window. After a time (and I do not know the exact amount of time) I take a few additional breaths and my hand is held over my heart, and then I touch her midshoulder on the back, and touch my heart at the same time.

Search

I am picking up info through a myriad of senses, those we call physical and those I call intuitive . . . knowing. I am deeply kinesthetic—a way of perceiving that I owned a long time ago. During this treatment I am immediately connected to her throat and her heart. My heart feels a flutter that I note is a fear or anxiety that R is living daily. I realize that she is fearful of the consequences of saying what is in her heart and I know that this is around her scholarly work.

The assessment proceeds in an ordered way. I move from crown to foot and return to areas where I want a bit more info. On this day I am redrawn to R's solar plexus area. I would describe it as sleeping, which I know sounds weird but that is what it is. I begin to wonder in a way if there is a bit of disconnect between upper and lower chakras . . . somehow intertwined with this throat-heart anxiety. I am also drawn to her shoulders and I immediately envision stone.

Rebalance

I begin with the intention of general relaxation . . . softening . . . opening . . . that she might be "more able" to receive the energy that moves through my being—my hands—and is offered to her. I use sweeping motions, generalized as it were . . . I envision the words "relax," "safe," and I say them silently. I use my hands to gently "massage" her stony shoulders and actually see them softening.

I feel in my being a release—that is how I would describe it, almost like a cleansing breath—and I know I am "shifting" (though I never thought of it in terms of my consciousness shifting). I move toward her heart space and my intention is to offer quietness, lessening anxiety because as I continue to work I am more clear that the anxiety is really getting in her way, really blocking her. With gentle, soft motions of my left hand while my right is on her left shoulder, I send quiet. I allow my hand movements to integrate her rhythm and as they are more rapid at first, they move toward slowing. During this time I become aware of a beautiful light-creamy pink coloring that is enfolding R.

Again I sense this feeling of readiness . . . release . . . and know it is time to continue. We have moved deeper into our shared experience with intention of reconnection. I begin but I am stopped and drawn to her solar plexus area, where I actually see a bright light that is not really colored, but not uncolored either. I know it is time to send energy through her adrenals, which I do by sharing that feeling I know from being in nature—not the sun necessarily, for me it is the energy of the natural world.

I next begin to work toward reconnection and rebalance of flow between R's higher centers . . . crown to brow to throat to heart . . . a stream of flowing, a gentle, continuous flow of movement. I am using hand motions and moving crown to foot in continuous sweeps that are ordered and rhythmic. I do not know how many minutes this goes on but I am aware at a point of R's even deeper breathing and she verbally releases—her head bends forward . . . I know that there is now a more connected flow. I am drawn to her back and I am standing. I actually rest her upon my lower abdomen and upper legs and she is peacefully there. I hold her shoulders, move a bit over her "chest," and support her rest. I complete her TT . . . I reassess, ground her.

Done

There is a shared shift. We both know that we are complete. She rests deeply for twenty minutes. I sit quietly.

What chakra do I use? I would say my crown and my heart direct my hands and my posture is flexible, relaxed.

When we are complete, I can tell by the way my being feels. It is another form of stillness . . . almost what I would call a peace and a completion in this moment.

Recall

I have dreams of this person. I cannot say they are at a particular frequency yet they occur, it seems, just when they are supposed to occur. The dreams are clear and we are together. I am aware that this is real connection . . . yes.

Often when I have these dreams I call or write to her. They seem, of late (over the last few years), to show up when she is in a space of discernment . . . not always an anxious space, but one I would term contemplative.

Case 15

Processing World War II

An elderly veteran struggles to find peace with his past.

Approach

T was smiling and there was an acceptance in his field.

Outreach

My hand chakras are assessing the field as I move my hands back and forth.

Search/Assessment

I am sensing differences in the energy field as I do the assessment starting from the head, moving down to the feet.

Rebalance

He is always lying on the daybed in their family room so I sit on a chair at the head of the daybed and move to his shoulders, and send comfort from my heart chakra. I then stand up, reassess the field, and end with grounding at the feet. T, eighty-five years old, was an assassin at Iwo Jima during WWII. He stated that he was unable to talk about his experiences for forty-five years, and now he can't stop talking about them. He talks constantly in very graphic detail through the treatment. This makes it challenging for me to stay on center during the treatment. My perception is that he needs to talk, and TT seems to give him permission to talk. There is always some sobbing during the talking.

Done

I sense calmness and relaxation and he seems to have come to the end of his stories. At the end of the session, T takes my hands to see if they are cold, because he felt a cool breeze over his body while I was working with him.

Recall

I think about his TT treatments. Even though his son says that he has seen a large change in his father in that his temperament is much calmer, I wonder if his treatments would be more beneficial if I didn't have to concentrate so much on returning to my center while I'm working with him. I have been treating him two or three times a month for two years.

<u>Case 16</u>

Taking Notes from the Inner Self:
Reviewing a Session

A therapist relates her process of reviewing a TT session with her Inner Self.

I sit down, paper and pencil in hand, and close my eyes to conference with my Inner Self. As usual, she has kept a nice file of her observations, including "video clips." However, her notes are not written in a linear, logical fashion. I must decipher them. She gets frustrated with me at times; to my Inner Self I must seem really obtuse.

She starts with a video clip, and time slows to a frame-by-frame pace as I see the treatments through her eyes. I observe that centering, which used to be a chore for me, now happens instantaneously. In slow motion I see a shift in the vibration in my physical body; an alignment and enlivening of my chakras. This alignment then extends to entrain with (plug into) the universal healing energies—from above, around, and deep into the earth. I ask to be a conduit for those energies, for whatever is in the greatest and highest good of the healee.

Approach

As I approach the healee, who is a friend of mine, we become surrounded by a golden-white light. My hand chakras begin to tingle slightly and come to full attention. In the notebook of my Inner Self she has suggested analogies—like a drug-sniffing dog just before being let off the leash to begin a search or a racehorse at the starting gate. (My Inner Self has a rich sense of humor, I think. Interesting analogies!) My hands begin.

Outreach

I make contact with the healee's shoulders, and my heart and hand chakras greet her Inner Self, sending love and peace. There is only this moment.

Search

The search begins and my hand chakras are on! (Inner Self notes say, "like a dog's ears pricking up when it hears something.") Cues come in many forms via hands, solar plexus, and heart. The healee takes a deep breath and immediately more flow happens in her field. Pain here; blockage here; stagnation here. Within me, the bloodhound's nose delivers the info. I get the taste that tells me the healee is undergoing chemo, and much of this can be moved out of the field.

Rebalance

As the rebalancing begins, my Inner Self shows me a short video clip. The physical bodies are essentially not visible in this clip, with the subtle energies clearly apparent. The moving colors of the two fields during the treatment are a beautiful, ethereal dance to watch. Back to the notes.

There is sadness, grief in the healee's heart area. Inner Self has gently guided my hands there. (Of course she can be two places at once!) I smooth the area and send love. And blue. Gently my hands continue to be directed by my third eye, the Inner Selves of both myself and the healee. Blockages are freed, flow continues down her legs, and what no longer serves her flows out the bottom of her feet into Mother Earth, where it will be converted for some other's benefit. Again the healee takes a deep cleansing breath and lets out a sigh. A tear slowly rolls down her cheek. It is a gift to walk this journey with this courageous woman. I am deeply honored.

The dance between search and rebalance continues. Soon I am holding her feet. How apt that I sit at the feet of the healee. My hands gently lift off her feet and move slightly to the side, palms facing her at a slight upward angle. *Anything else?* my Inner Self inquires of hers. Ahhh, the two Inner Selves are congruent.

Done

By mutual agreement the session is done. I gently scoot farther out of her field and sit with her until she opens her eyes. She smiles. I offer her water, a couch, and a blanket.

As Inner Self and I continue to look through her files, I come to understand that the search and rebalance described above is a collection of info concerning a week's worth of treatments of my friend who has been recently diagnosed with cholangiocarcinoma. Other aspects are parts of many treatments from September through December, 2011. A total of eighteen treatments are enfolded into this writing.

I make a cup of tea and sit down at the computer to write this. Reviewing the original documents, I see I missed an area. Recall. For this, Inner Self tells me, I am on my own. So . . . the final area to be addressed:

Recall

It is a regular part of my TT practice to treat people who have cancer. Since I see them frequently over a fairly long period of time, I often have dreams that involve that person. Sometimes the information is quite clear, such as a need to phone the person or to suggest a certain CD for her. I may get clear info (and this often comes during the treatment itself) that the healee needs something in particular, for example, to drink more water. Or to take a particular supplement, or eat more of a particular food. Other times, I have to sit with the dream in meditation to see if meaning unfolds. And at times, if there is meaning, it might be too obscure for me in that form. This can happen not only during sleeping dreams, but also during meditation, or sometimes just during a quiet moment.

One time I kept getting "dates" for a healee who had cancer. Dates, dates, dates. Hmmm. A calendar? A new relationship? No—the fruit! I looked them up and found that those dates have been shown to shrink cancerous tumors. Aha.

My Inner Self—like me, I think—rarely sleeps.

Case 17
Resonating with Nursing Home Residents

This case was done in a seventy-five-bed nursing home where many of the residents have dementia. TT has been offered here for more than twenty years and has been incorporated into policies and procedures for both Nursing and Life Enrichment. Staff have noted both calming of agitation and improved sleep for residents after TT "moments." And when staff receive TT, they report reduced stress and muscle aches.

Approach

I begin each session by first making sure that I am "rooted," as Dora expresses it. This involves my root chakra—a feeling of being here on Earth for an earthly purpose, not "so heavenly minded that I am no earthly good," as my mother used to say. Once grounded and beginning the session, I am no longer aware of the root chakra involvement; it hums along in the background unnoticed. I also am aware of my solar plexus chakra in the sense that I feel that this is my life task, that I have the knowledge and capability to do healing. I feel confident as I approach the session, and this I think comes from my solar plexus. This also hums along in the background; I don't feel it as being involved in the same way as the higher chakras.

If I don't know the person, I always take a hand and introduce myself. Immediately my heart chakra responds to this contact and I can usually see a relaxation in the healee's whole body. Often I receive impressions of the healee's emotions—fear, sadness, and so on. I speak softly, and gently introduce the concept of Therapeutic Touch. My throat chakra also seems to be involved at this point—perhaps as I feel the connection through my heart.

I then center. For me centering involves becoming aware, through my hand chakras, of the rhythm of my own field. As I do this there's a shift in consciousness and the crown chakra is immediately involved, followed by the throat chakra. At this point I feel my connection to my Inner Self. This connection remains throughout as long as I remain deeply centered. If I lose this deep center, I can return to it quickly by consciously becoming aware of the rhythm of the field. As I center, feeling the resonance between my hands, and with my intention to help restore order to the field of my healing partner, I often note a relaxation response in the patient right at that moment.

Outreach

Each session is unique. In all cases I am led by the field of my healing partner, supporting him in his own healing. The session unfolds as it will. Since I center through my hand chakras, they are feeling the rhythm of my field. As I go into the assessment I do the traditional assessment/scan of the field—my hands are deep listening, noting differences in the field such as heat/cold/texture/imbalances. This is my ritual stage. I am aware of my heart chakra being connected to that of my healing partner, and then my crown chakra engages. At this point my hands are already starting the assessment, and if the relaxation response has not already been noted, it is now.

Search and Rebalance

At this point I begin to consciously go deeper to work with the rhythm of the field. Immediately I feel a stronger pulsing in my crown chakra and it seems to connect inside my head with the third eye. At the same time, my heart chakra is involved. I often, at this point, feel a sense of unition with the healing partner, Inner Self, and the universal healing field. Then my throat chakra is involved as well.

I assess the rhythm of the field in a pattern. My right hand (usually I am on the person's left side, but if space requires it, my left hand works equally well) starts above the head and moves down the spine, resonating with the healing partner's field. Where there is a disruption in the rhythm, my hand usually pauses and gently pulses there until the healing partner's field begins to resonate with it. This may take several minutes and several passes through the field. If it is difficult to get resonance, I stop and do some unruffling in the area, and then return to the resonating passes until our fields are in full resonance there. While doing this, my left hand is placed just beyond the healee's feet [the patient is supine], assessing whether the energy is coming through well or not.

When working with the rhythm I am also "listening" and often hear notes (soul notes?) that I use to help with the resonance. If I am in a place where I can sing without being thought weird or crazy, then I sing the note out loud. Sometimes I am moved to sing a series of notes with different vowel sounds. At the nursing home I may be moved to sing an old hymn that seems to aid with the resonance. At these times the throat chakra is actively working and pulsing. I typically sing it inside my head, if not out loud, to aid in the resonance.

I continue to assess and balance the field by moving my hand down each side of the spine, then each arm, working to create resonance as described earlier. While working with the rhythm I often become momentarily unaware of any separation among myself, the healing partner, Inner Self, and the universal healing field. I become the vibration, setting up a resonating field with that of my healing partner. This, I think, originates from the order of the healing field and my connection to that field through Inner Self. I meet the Inner Self of my healing partner there and together we "dance" to the vibration of the universal healing field, moving through the various levels of consciousness. At each level of consciousness we respond with a resonating field, facilitating a return to an ordered, balanced state.

Done

How do I know that the TT treatment is completed? I know that the treatment is finished when my hands move through all areas of the healing partner's field in resonance with my own field. I get a deep sense of satisfaction and a sense that we have completed our healing dance.

Recall

I don't connect with the healees in recollection. I find this odd, since I do have a deep connection when I am working with them. I do, sometimes, get a nudge to give someone a Therapeutic Touch session. I always try to follow up on these hunches and get feedback. Usually there is a good reason for having done the TT.

Case 18
Surrender Near the End of Life

A therapist supports a healee over a long battle with cancer.

Approach

As W and I walk together to the treatment room, I sense what could be described as a mixture of feelings—fear, joy, sadness (profound, breathtaking sadness), confusion, courage. If I could say this it feels almost like all these feeling states plus more are almost competing for top priority. I am still, quiet, breathing deeply as I call upon my inner resources to stand with me. As she shares her journey of living with cancer for fifteen years, expressing itself in a variety of locations within her, I know in the deepest part of my being that she is moving within and will soon make her transition. How do I know that? I just do. And I know as well that she knows it too, and at least part of her struggle is living with peace. She has been and continues to be a fighter—how does surrendering to the reality of what is speak to the internal fighter? She sits quietly . . . I feel still and ready.

Outreach

As we walk together we do not hold hands but one of my arms is behind her and I am deeply aware that her solar plexus is rumbling! Isn't that just it? We talk . . . and hold hands . . . and proceed.

Search

I am immediately drawn to her solar plexus and I sense swirling—there is a disorder, a need to scream, to cry, to laugh . . . laugh? I question that and recheck . . . yes, to laugh. I see her gripping a tin roof . . . slipping, holding. I sense she desires freedom—the freedom of letting go, flying as it were on the wings of the wind . . . but something . . . no someone . . . is holding her. It is her holding her—intertwined with others whom she loves deeply. This swirling is born from this, at least in part.

I continue seeking, assessing, and am struck by her deep courage. There is a beautiful flower—it is golden and the blooms are full. It is a flower that closes in the twilight. I sense that W's twilight is upon her. As I continue my assessment, discovering . . . when I am near her crown I see movement in a variety of directions . . . movement without rhythm, confusion. How do I know? I can see it in my mind's eye. As I continue I actually feel the emptiness . . . yes, I am centered . . . yes, of course I check that out . . . yes.

Rebalance

I had been immediately drawn to her solar plexus and I sense swirling—my hands begin to move in smoother rhythmic "waves" that begin here and ultimately move toward the ground. My intention is to quiet the swirling, and in the quiet, the deeper need will manifest for her. I am not holding expectations. As we continue this her tears become a sob. I move to her heart and gently hold it; I enfold her in blue—a deep Dora blue—and open space for her release. The sobs intensify; I continue to hold. Her body almost jerks, which I realize is good; it is a release, almost a freeing. I have no idea of the time but we continue until I sense a profound and deepening stillness.

I then continue, and it is now that I am more aware of her core strength moving crown to foot and beyond—straight, steady, solid. I feel this and I think I might have even stood straighter (I am not sure). I move my hands in gentle ordered motions with the intention of supporting, sustaining this.

Done

I sense a "lightening-ness" and I know this treatment is complete. She rests for fifteen minutes. I sit quietly.

Recall

I next saw W in December when she came to the TT group practice sessions. We exchanged a look of deep knowing that I am at this moment having trouble finding words to describe. She was treated by another therapist. Afterward, during our therapist debriefing, the practitioner (my student) shared her experience. She shared that when she treated W she "could not feel her field" and sensed that she was going to die soon.

This opened up an opportunity for our group to share thoughts on "fields in transition." And it offered us, as well, the opportunity to collectively quiet our minds and send W thoughts of peace.

Editor's Note: Follow-Up

In reflection several years later, the TT therapist recalled that it was about two weeks after this final meeting that W made her transition. It was a winter day with a very heavy snowfall, which prevented our therapist from going to see W one last time. She retains a clear memory across the years: "I remember so clearly enfolding us both in peace and calling for help from my not physically present helpers." This eloquently speaks to the timeless space we experience in Therapeutic Touch.

The Healing Dance

Rather than submitting a single case study with one individual, this long-time TT therapist shared a narrative reflecting her personal approach, both as a healer and a healee. Her account is a beautiful illustration of how we sometimes dance between the two roles.

Approach

In my role as healer I start with the familiar, inquiring about comfort (physical and otherwise) while sensing and responding to both verbal and nonverbal cues ("Is it okay for me to come closer now? Are you comfortable, physically and otherwise?"). I see this phase as the energy equivalent of shaking hands—a reaching out to the other, assessing/testing whether I will be invited to step across the threshold. It also may involve my answering questions, both asked and sensed.

Outreach

This flows, apparently seamlessly, from the familiar process of introducing myself to gaining access to the healee with the intention of helping/healing. This also seems to be a transition time from what is familiar to the healee, and what may be new. Relaxation takes place during this phase (and continues through the TT process).

My process as healer is to consciously relax, take deep breaths, and center with palms up as I await a sense of connection and feel the flow of compassion, search for the information that will guide my hands.

Note: If centering is interrupted [by external circumstances or wandering thoughts], the centering process may be repeated as needed, since the TT process takes place from/within a centered state.

Search

At some point during outreach, search begins. Hands, which have been stroking the field, are waiting for the energetic invitation to "see" further, and for cues/differences (for me, usually vague at this point, known more to my hands than to my brain).

This is the foundation for the beginning of the TT: permission to be in the field/to see or know and to help restore wholeness and balance. This represents an implicit contract to help and to heal. It is important to use the word "heal" with care, lest it be interpreted as cure. The outcome is not in our hands.

As my hands start to move gently in the field, I transition from verbal to predominantly nonverbal; from focus on the physical expanding to encompassing the entire human energy field. Respirations of both healer and healee grow slower and deeper, shoulders start to relax.

Note: I used to hear others discuss in great detail what they "saw," and feel I wasn't there yet. Over time I have come to believe that I will sense/see what is needed in order to help that person at that time. My expectation is not what I can do, rather how I can be used to help/heal. This belief was strengthened during an interaction at Pumpkin Hollow Farm when a pregnant friend asked me to treat her. I initially declined; never having treated a pregnant mother, I had concerns for the fetus. She reassured me that it was because of my concern/awareness that she was asking me. During assessment I held the intention that the TT was for Mom, and invited the baby to take what it wanted or needed. I had a very clear insight, almost like a drawing in an anatomy book, that I was treating her muscles alongside the vertebrae, and that the energy was flowing around, not through, her uterus—while the fetus was safe and comfortable in its own space.

Rebalance

Again there is a flow, more circular than linear. During treatment it seems that assessment and treatment are in the same time frame, rather than a linear sequence (although the latter is really helpful in teaching new students).

Done

Consciousness shifts back to present time/place, accompanied by the feeling to offer the healee a sense of grounding by placing my hands on the feet. (While doing this, I often see the image of a tree rooted firmly and securely in the earth.) This is accompanied by a transition from the atemporal, aspatial consciousness I experience during treatment to the physical present. I remove my hands from the feet, observe the healee (back in 3D!) and inquire if he/she is ready to move to a comfortable place to rest. I typically sit quietly, gradually bringing my attention fully back to my physical surroundings. When the healee is ready to transition from resting, I am waiting nearby to assist. Feedback varies, following rest, and if/when the healee wishes.

Recall

I have been able to shift consciousness during recall of TT, atemporal and aspatial from the 1980s or 2000s—it seems that TT memories are polydimensional, accessible by having or recalling actual, similar, or parallel experiences. (In both words and action in TT we enter a universe described/perceived as atemporal, aspatial, and multidimensional. Yet my vocabulary doesn't seem adequate for the concepts I am attempting to describe.)

Notes: The effort of *trying* can interfere with the process of TT, which benefits from letting go and letting it flow, trusting that the energy will know. This both supports and emphasizes Dora's admonition to TT practitioners to "Set the ego aside!"

Apologia: I have not had a regular practice during this time period, having been in both the healer and healee roles. I will note the TT sessions I did give: to a friend with a back injury, another with a stroke, a third who was widowed this year, a woman I met in Florida who had recent back surgery, and a hospital patient as requested by her room-mate (my friend). In some cases I also did TT with friends or family members of several healees, typically requested after observing my offering TT to the initial healee.

There were also instances of experiencing TT as both healee and healer while in Montana at Dee's annual Dialogues gatherings. Being offered the experience as healee let me experience the notion of TT as mutual process, tremendously strengthened by experiencing it as healer-healee; I continue to learn so much from both. (I suspect my mind is only privy to one or two of the multiple dimensions involved with this mystical/practical process.)

Blessings and gratitude to Dee for having the heart, the intellect, and the courage to share/promote/teach and support the development and dissemination of Therapeutic Touch.

Three Decades of TT Inform Daily Interactions

A therapist reviews her thirty-year commitment to Therapeutic Touch as a way of life.

From my perspective in describing my experiences with TT looking over my shoulder, TT is more than a therapeutic session with a client; the practice informs my daily interactions. The experience can be compared to the difference between meditation as a seated posture and meditation as continuous mindfulness. Based on my three decades of invaluable TT training, Therapeutic Touch—as Dee poignantly expressed—is a way of life.

The treasured tools of Therapeutic Touch serve me as a spiritual heightening of my sensibilities to engage subtle energies within each being, energies beyond our five senses that comprise the essential essence of our true nature.

Grounded in clarity, acting with compassion and the intention to be an instrument of healing, each interaction with others becomes an awareness of our unity, not our otherness. Our skin, in myriad shapes and colors, is not limitation-bound but permeable evanescence through which flows a vital-energy stream.

Essential to each TT session is profound appreciation and respect for the person or people engaged in the therapeutic exchange. The silent dialogue, or dance to promote healing, always acknowledges the mutual freedom implicit in the encounter. There is constant recognition that all souls—healing partners—know what is best for them in alignment with intended purpose.

The presence of freedom is palpable with no expectations of outcomes or cure. The unified experience culminating any TT interaction is firmly grounded in self-knowledge by the individuated self, who immediately perceives any projections or identification. Beyond separate but equal I find connected and mutual.

In the therapeutic exchange one enters the experience with understanding of our shared humanity, discernment without judgment. Signals are picked up by the tingling hands, warmth or its absence, blockage or release, but the need for rebalance is made conscious through each relevant chakra corresponding to the situation. Completion for me is indicated by blue light in the third eye and a centered sense of wholeness and well-being intuitively felt as harmony and peacefulness.

Love not as an emotion but as a state of being permeates the energetic field. The word "unconditional" is inappropriate, for the dynamic transcends conditions. The radiance of light and bliss fulfill and complete the TT interaction.

I conclude by conveying my abiding appreciation for the art and science of Therapeutic Touch, the blessing, which transforms my way of being in the world.

On Significant Experiential Factors during Each Phase

Included here in this abridged version of "Looking Over My Shoulder" are Dolores Krieger's own responses, in which she identifies herself as DEEK.

Search

I am centered. I feel rooted and grounded. In the aura of protection of my Inner Self I am open, alert, and aware, and sense the permission to allow my sensitivities full range.

There is a sense of undisturbed weightlessness, and in this environment of pure calm, my concentration deepens. My perceptions sharpen and pictures float across my mind as I establish a deeper relationship with my healing partner.

Memories well up—Aha! I am aware of sensations of consciousness from the chakras in the vital-energy field overlying my hands. Slight changes in my healing partner's personal energy, cues from energetic movements and tone, shifts in rhythm, unexpected variations of scintillating colors—all register in my mind as objective, unbiased sensory data.

Identify more closely with my healing partner and, lo, I'm in a timeless space! I am conscious of subtle perceptions—clear, though altered states of consciousness. The overriding compassion that I feel for the healing partner becomes tinged with awe and sheer joy. I feel a sense of anticipation from the healing partner and I am aware of the power of our rapport. This sense of oneness evokes feelings of reverence for the deep self we share—an ineffable state. Words fail me.

Approach

As I turn my attention to the healing partner, I realize that I am shifting the focus of my state of consciousness to my "within." In fact, a number of shifts happen simultaneously or with an almost imperceptible lag time.

My gaze foreshortens, my respiratory rate becomes slower and deeper, a deep "listening" state is available, and I notice that my hand and heart chakras have "turned on." I can still see as I normally do; however, my visual field seems to have shifted focus and I seem to be short-sighted, the focal point somewhere behind my physical eyes, while simultaneously my sight is coming from a palpable area about two to three inches in front of the midpoint of my forehead. As I get more deeply into this state, frequently (increasingly so in the past few years) visualizations occur about the healing partner's condition. My intuition seems to be linked to the visualizations.

My throat chakra, of which I'm not usually aware, seems to be actively functioning. There seems to be a calm, steady background of awareness that comes from, or includes, both the solar plexus and the throat chakras. However, the major chakra that is strongly (rhythmically) and constantly functioning on many levels of consciousness is the heart chakra.

A strong bond of compassion links me to the healing partner and I am aware that my crown-ajna chakras are functioning.

It is out of this compendium of subtle functions that I know where to lightly place my hand chakras, on or just beyond the periphery of the healing partner's physical body.

Outreach and Search

Outreach and search seem to work together as a state of consciousness and simultaneously slide out of approach as the approach state culminates. This simultaneity continues as below; however, some subtle boundary conditions remain (so the outreach and search phases do not form a true continuum).

As I put my hand chakras into the healing partner's fields, I deep-listen more intently and feel the differences in his fields.

Information flows in very quickly as I explore the differentiated areas.

The information is frequently supplemented by moments of clear visualization coupled with intuitive flashes.

The healing partner's fields become more perceptible to my hand chakras, particularly his psychodynamic field, and I feel what is in imbalance. I also may have strong emotional reactions to the uptake of information.

I often sense a presence, which I associate with my Inner Self, that feels like an overshadowing. It seems to be a familiar feeling and I feel at peace with it and can go on with the work at hand.

The patterns of subtle energies that I feel reveal more information to me. As I direct my sensitivities to these patterned areas, I get a clearer sense of what is in imbalance, traumatized, and so on. Other variables, such as dysrhythmias or change in the texture or in the subtle luminescence of the field, are also important indicators.

Particularly in conjunction with visualization, I often get a sense of the origin of the healing partner's problem or condition.

The heart, ajna, and crown chakras seem most active during this phase of the TT process, with the throat chakra often coming into play, and the throat chakra sometimes becoming active.

Rebalance

Depending upon my assessment, or an obvious need, initial efforts are concerned with:

- Modulating the healing partner's energy.
- Directing the pranic flow from the universal healing field.
- Projecting my own energy, or otherwise sharing energy, as in scaffolding.
- Later in the TT session, on an as-needed basis, I may shift to a Deep Dee.
- My sense of it is that I am working closely with Inner Self during this time. I occasionally sense angelic or other presences during rebalancing, though this may also happen earlier in the TT treatment.
- Once I have the details out of the way, I try to have my personality stand aside by concentrating and visualizing the living radiance of Inner Self projecting through my heart, ajna, and particularly the crown chakras flowing to the healing partner. Keeping my deep-listening functions available to Inner Self, I maintain a sense of stillness and let the prana flow through me to the healing partner.

Done

There are several indicants:

- The pranic flow lessens.
- I can see that the healing partner is in relaxation response and may be sleeping.

- The healing partner gets restless, uncomfortable, fatigues, or experiences pain (due to TT treatment).
- Information inflow lessens.
- The partner feels "cooked" to me, and my sense is that he has had enough of the TT interaction.
- Most usually he then sleeps for a while, and I let him self-awaken.

Recall

- I rarely remember dreams. However, many years ago I was startled out of a deep sleep by a visualization that a patient was in the hospital in severe trouble. I woke, drove to the hospital, and ran to the patient's room where she, a quadriplegic, was dying of suffocation. She was connected to a respirator; inadvertently the porter had pulled the electric plug out of the socket as he left the room, unaware of what he had done.
- I am very sensitive to a healing partner's needs and seem to be checking him out telepathically or visualizing him during meditation or reverie. Occasionally I visualize him intentionally. At those times I seem to be standing next to or near him.
- If there is a problem, I'm most often aware of it.
- Very frequently I'll be thinking of a person and within a short time that person phones or emails me.

Post TT Session Comments
The following comments were reported by DEEK and her healing partner respectively, following a session.

Healing Partner

- I was in abject pain; it (low back) really hurt. Surprisingly quickly, as the TT session began, the core of the pain released. I felt myself let loose a deep breath, as though the held breath were liberated, no longer bound in my chest.
- Shortly thereafter I felt myself more psychologically and psychically integrated. The feelings of pain became more coherent. It felt like

the "chunk" of pain broke down into segments, and I could get a hold of it; that is, be in control of the situation.

- Now the pain is much less, barely perceptible, and I feel in control. I even remember what I wanted when I came back into this room. Thank you; I'd almost forgotten what that (short-term memory) felt like.

DEEK

- As I approached the healing partner I felt a definite difference of frequency, rhythm, and texture—the "feel" of her pranic flow—from my own.

- I was aware of a meshing of our subtle fields as I neared her. I tried to "get in" farther or more deeply, felt a resistance, and eased off somewhat. I did this emotionally by identifying with her less intensely, giving over to Inner Self, and physically by withdrawing a bit, shifting the rhythm of my breathing, using my hand chakras to "unruffle" her subtle fields. I noted I was becoming more objective.

- With that shift in consciousness I felt an uplifting exchange of pranic flow between us. I waited to feel that flow in each area of her fields in which I was engaged. I kept my hands moving lightly. Finally I felt it was okay to bring my hand chakras gently over her solar plexus, and then over her heart chakra. Almost immediately I felt a relaxation response in the partner.

- I focused on my own crown chakra, did a Deep Dee check on her, and then projected TT blue to her thalamic area from my heart chakra-crown flow. Her relaxation response seemed to deepen. I rechecked her, let her sleep, and went out of the room.

8

Healing-at-a-Distance
Exploratory Study

In its original form, as developed during the mid-twentieth century, TT is done in the presence of the healing partner, the healee, while the healer works therapeutically in the healee's pranic fields. The present study is based on an intensive questionnaire that delves into the TT therapist's sense of interiority as she proceeds through the healing process at a distance.

The sample size of this exploratory study was forty Therapeutic Touch therapists, each of whom had at least three years' experience with the TT process. The format of the questionnaire follows the healer's engagement of the healing-at-a-distance process from its beginning until the end of the session. In addition to an in-depth analysis and discussion of the responses to the questionnaire, a summary of the study's major conclusions and recommendations for future studies are offered.

Although healing at-a-distance has an ancient history, most often it has been practiced as an article of faith within religious settings. It is only within the past few decades that validating studies have demonstrated scientific authenticity. Since then, there has been a significant increase of interest in this manner of remote healing that has attracted professional attention, notably in the fields of the biosciences, social studies, and the health sciences. Physicists Russell Targ and Harold Puthoff are just two of the researchers into this area. Their work demonstrates what TT therapists have always felt—that time and space can become irrelevant in the realms of human interaction.

From the Theoretical to the Practical: Steps in Healing at-a-Distance

Healing at-a-distance is an act of interiority; in the present study the term is used to denote a personal process of working with prana (vital energy) with the intent of helping or healing a person or situation physically removed from the healer.

There were 268 item responses from forty active respondents to this questionnaire. Thirty-eight of the entire sample of forty healers used a Therapeutic Touch healing-at-a-distance healing style. The following is the basic form of TT healing at-a-distance.

As the healer begins the healing session:

- She maintains a state of sustained centering throughout the healing session.
- She seeks out and communicates with her Inner Self.
- She visualizes the healing partner; that is, rather than imagining a representation of the individual, the healer clearly visualizes herself near the healee.
- She checks the validity of her visualization; she sensitively visualizes that space so that she now has a clear idea of where the person is in relation to the door and window(s) of his room.
- She sensitizes herself to the healing partner's pranic streams, and simultaneously listens deeply to any communication from her own Inner Self.
- On the basis of these sensory cues she decides upon a treatment plan for modulating and directing prana to meet the needs of the healee.
- When there is no further incoming information about the healing partner, the healer often does a final reassessment before ending the session.

Participants' Responses

In the Beginning

The Call: What Is the First Thing You Do?

Responses varied among the TT therapists. For the majority, the first thing chosen was among the following:

- Engage in sustained centering
- Take a deep breath
- Become physically comfortable
- Close my eyes
- Visualize the healing partner
- Listen deeply

Briefly describe the first thing that you do when you answer a call to do healing at-a-distance for someone who is ill.

Therapists describe a range of things they do to prepare for a healing-at-a-distance session, running the gamut from simple administrative details to preparations for deep interior work:

- *∅* I set the time for the healing interaction to take place, such as before, during, or after the healee's surgery, or when he is asleep or napping.
- *∅* I make sure I will not be disturbed during the TT treatment.
- *∅* I breathe deeply to reduce my desires re personal outcome.
- *∅* I simply wait very quietly for a visual image to appear. This signals the connection between the healing partner and me.
- *∅* I begin by scanning my own field to identify my own emotions (about the healing session).
- *∅* I seek out what is best for the client.
- *∅* I ask to serve as an instrument of healing.
- *∅* I sometimes simply visualize the healee's name as if written on a chalkboard and know that healing energy is going to him with my intention.

I set my intent to be of service and restore order, balance, and harmony to the field. I see the client as perfect, whole, and complete—the wholeness in me reaching out to the wholeness in my healing partner. I maintain a loving and compassionate attitude.

Perception of Self

Where do you see yourself? Do you visualize the location in your mind's eye? Do you see yourself with the healing partner?

- Usually I have a sense of having traveled to the other person.
- I usually go in spirit. I leave my physical body behind and see my whole body there in spirit with the person.
- I see the healee in front of me and I can actually feel/perceive his energy field and do a treatment as if he were physically in front of me.
- I visualize gently approaching the healing partner, introducing myself, explaining why I am there and the general procedure. I make sure he understands that he is in charge and can stop the session at any time if desired.
- I take myself to the healee and feel and see myself with him or her. Most of the time I am upstairs in a chair and I am "beside" the healee.
- I am lightly aware of my physical body in its physical location . . . I go to be present with the healee nonphysically.
- I am aware of where I am at physically, but I have also connected in another time dimension with the healee so I am also with him.
- I'm generally in the same position(s) I would be in if we were physically together.
- I'm usually standing or sitting by the healing partner, but many times several feet away.
- During my visualizations I feel that I am standing right in front of (or behind) the individual, just as if I were there in person. I am looking from my eyes and can see my hands and arms.

Are you "assisted" energetically by other beings? Are you aware of nonhelpful presences? How do you distinguish other beings

from the energies of the patient, visitors, Inner Self, or others? Are the beings connected to or associated with the healee, or are they familiar guides, presences for the TT practitioner?

- I have a sense when someone (in the room) is already full of loving energy toward the healing partner and there is a connection.
- I have occasionally had a sense of other beings supporting the process, and there are times when I feel drawn to asking the healee's angels, archangels, and supportive beings to assist with the process. There is a sense of the process being enhanced by these supportive beings.
- Other beings are instantly available when I call upon them; usually they speak in my mind. They are familiar presences, very loving and helpful.
- As in an in-person healing, this healing session is between the patient and me only. The exception is if higher aspects of the patient make their presence felt.
- There are often guides and other entities to help me on the journey and to support the healing.
- I can sense other beings' presence sometimes.
- I like to call upon the devic healing forces for help, and Raphael the Archangel of Healing at times.
- Recently, especially when doing distance healing on persons requested through our TT group, I have sensed the presence of others' energies available in this space and helping with the healing.

As you connect with the healee's energy, do you experience yourself more energetically than as a physical form? If so, do you experience any difficulty in returning to full waking consciousness in your physical self?

- My physical form is as though I am an essence, and often my mind's screen is filled with light that is usually white or blue-white.
- There are times when I feel I am in a meditative state and energy is moving through and from me to the healee. Other times it is as if my physical being is pure energy so there is no me sitting on the

chair in this location; my energy meets the energy of the healee somewhere and we interact with each other.

- Our energies meet somewhere that is undefinable.

- I see the patient in front of me and I can actually feel/perceive his energy field and do a TT as if he were physically in front of me. Many times I get visual images surrounding things I am picking up in the field.

- In my mind and heart I go to be present with the client nonphysically by visualizing him or invoking his energy through his name. I am mostly aware of being present with the client's energy signature.

- It's as if my consciousness is present with the healing partner at the same time as I am in this different time dimension. It's like the inside of the universe where there is no separation of time and space.

- I am no longer present in my body. I am energy only.

- I don't see myself at all. It is more a sense of the healing partner's rhythm that will flow through a sense of my own rhythm. At first the two rhythms are a bit of a distance apart. Then during assessment and treatment there is more focus on the healee, so I'm only noticing his rhythm(s) and at times possibly a blurring of rhythms with an awareness of the healee's dysrhythms in contrast to my rhythm. This sounds more linear and concrete than my actual experience. It is fluid and more like being in currents of waves.

- I go to be present with the patient by visualizing him.

- When the recipient is a stranger I see him only vaguely, as a nondescript figure in a grayish-white fog. When I feel a sense of connection with someone, such as with a TT friend whom I have met, I see the person much more clearly and feel as though I can talk with him.

- Sometimes I get very vivid images, and this is not usual for me. Once I was doing distance TT and in my mind's eye I saw a zipper open in the healee's left abdominal area, and then a whole pile of ants came scurrying out.

- I see colors and visions of textures depending on the area of body affected and sometimes for no reason. For example, I may see a white fuzziness in the abdominal area.

Sense of Place

Do you perceive the healee's environment? Do you have a sense of other persons, furniture, or instruments in the environment? Nonphysical beings or energies? What kind of atmosphere do you feel during the healing process? Examples might include light, radiance, upliftment, sounds, silence, or something else.

- On occasion I may have images of things in a room but usually have not had a way to validate whether they are real or imaginary.

- There is a deep quiet that feels as though I am basking in that silence . . . as if within the quiet "all is perceived." There is no effort; the information comes quickly and easily.

- I feel a sense of timelessness and of being connected to the whole. I feel a wonderful sense of unity and an openness.

- It is a lovely "place" to be and I do feel uplifted as I return to ordinary life. The place is wordless, silent, calm, and softly enveloping of me.

- I feel centered, compassionate, and sometimes empathic toward the person who requested the healing, and optimistic.

- The place is one of deep stillness. It's just me and the recipient and I usually don't hear distractions around me. I have this "aura of quietude" around me. Almost another dimension.

- A place of quiet, peace, wholeness, a "space" where there is only connection and love. It is closer to a deep silence, connectedness.

- I feel as if my healing partner and I are enveloped in a quiet, white space somewhere outside of my normal perception.

- My sense is we are meeting in a place out of space and time, in a void, pregnant with possibilities.

- Sometimes I have a sense that I am visiting the client on an astral level or in a lucid dream where we are both in an altered state of consciousness. Other times it seems like a telepathic connection on the physical level.

- I may see an angelic figure (in color and usually above the healing partner).

- Often I experience energetic allies in the room helping me when I'm doing distance healing. Though once I had a sense of the doctor coming into the healee's room and I stopped (his wife later verified).

- I get the feeling through the healing partner of other people and how they are responding to his illness at times.

Olfactory Sensations

Do you smell flowers, perfume, or other perceptible scents?

- Occasionally during meditation I smell roses or vanilla, or sometimes warm pine sap, but not generally during the actual distance treatment.

- I am not aware of any specific scent, but my breathing is deeper and I may associate an image with a scent—something from my memory, rather than something occurring during the session.

- I have detected fragrances while encountering a presence, but not when doing healing at-a-distance.

- On rare occasions I may smell a pipe, but that is a sign that a specific spirit is with me.

- Sometimes I would describe it as sweet rather than a flower or perfume. I sometimes get baking smells—cake or muffins.

- I have detected sweet-smelling flowers or perfume during the rest as I sit with a client, but not as a background for distance sessions.

- Whatever is in the environment of the healee. For example, if he is near water, the smell of the water.

Sounds Heard

Are there sounds heard as if with the ear, inner ear, or sensed? Do they come unbidden or are they specifically sought? Do they convey information, and if so, directly or symbolically?

- "Sight" and "sound" are not of the five senses, though occasionally a voice may provide a message for a loved one. (An example was a message about a sudden death: "It was a job well done and it is complete.") Sometimes there is succinct information to be conveyed to the patient, always in a constructive, supportive, and loving tone.

- Sometimes information comes in the form of thoughts documenting what is going on or what is needed to be done.

- I have heard words such as "done" when the session is finished. "No one is home" when the session is not to take place at that time.

- I hear voices from time to time. Sometimes they make me aware of the emotions felt by the recipient and the reason for the way he is feeling. Sometimes I've been told to hover a bit longer.

- It is not so much a separate "voice" that I "hear," but information or knowing that occurs; it may be a lot of information or a pithy sentence relating to the person. It sometimes feels like a download of information that is spoken in my head.

- I've speculated that the musical tone is an F#, but I've never been near an instrument to test that when it happens.

- I sometimes hear a voice say a word, but it is more in my head than in my ears.

- There is a sound I have heard in the background of my mind on and off for forty years. Have you ever been swimming in the ocean with the surf breaking on rocks and sand? Have you ever been underwater listening to the sounds between one wave and the next? When I am in a very good state spiritually, I can sometimes hear a faint hissing, rushing, tinkling sound, deep in the background of my mind, reminiscent of the sounds I've described above. Were it not for the high frequency components, I would say it sounds somewhat like a large, powerful waterfall in a creek. I have often interpreted this sound as being the audible life stream. However, I have no real knowledge of its origin. In any case, if I am really centered and have a solid footing energetically and things are flowing for me, I sometimes hear this sound while doing distance TT.

Memory

Do any experiences remind you of an incident in your life, a friend, a mood, or other memories?

- Sometimes visualizations spontaneously occur of an imaginative nature, which culminate in unity of a transcendent nature with the recipient. When described afterward to that person, the content has been reported to have resonance for him.
- I can relate to the patient's experience through my own experience of it.
- The calm, peaceful feeling is one I associate with lovely spiritual experiences or meditations I have had.
- Occasionally a previous experience when I was doing bedside nursing, and also when I felt the need for hope when my husband was on death's door.
- What I see first is the mood of the person and how this is affecting his health. I deal with his Inner Self, which is always joyful, and then we both work at the health problem. I sometimes talk to the healing partner and tell him it's okay to be healthy and to let the rest go.

Mind-to-Mind Communication

Do you feel you are in mind-to-mind communication when you are doing at-a-distance healing? What does heart-to-heart communication feel like; is there a physical aspect to it? How is it different from mind-to-mind communication?

- More heart-to-heart than mind-to-mind.
- I sometimes talk to the client in my mind and feel I am heard; no answers, just a feeling. Sometimes words well up from my heart and I feel the connection heart-to-heart.
- I feel an energetic connection with the healing partner and also an emotional connection. I don't really feel mind-to-mind, more a feeling of heart-to-heart.
- I feel in communication with my partner's whole being at an energetic level.
- I occasionally feel as though the patient is dimly aware of me, as you might be aware of someone coming into your bedroom while you are asleep. Once in a while I experience the sense that we have made a momentary conscious contact.

- Sometimes I know things that I do not know how I know. I am not directly aware, but assume these intelligences are communicating with my Inner Self.
- Sometimes I feel others are helping me; I once felt that another pair of hands was working with me.

Awareness of a Presence

Do you feel a sense of presence during the healing-at-a-distance session? How do you "know" the presence is there? How are you aware of different levels of consciousness; all at once or in sequence? What is the role of trust in the process? What is the role of faith? What is the role of music, harmonics, vibratory components?

- Connecting to my Inner Self, there is a feeling of *open sesame* and access to a larger presence.
- I have spirit guides that I use in TT, but I haven't really called on them when I do distance healing.
- They are in attendance as a silent presence so far.
- I always feel that I am the instrument and not the source, so there is a constant presence in my life of "the other."
- I feel an energetic type of presence during the session.
- From the answers I keep giving, I wonder if I go into a space that is beyond perception, but then don't have words to communicate it.
- I usually feel a sense of the presence of the recipient. Occasionally I also feel a deeper-than-normal sense of myself.
- Often I see different colors of light that change during the session.

Success of Treatment

How do you sense whether the healing at-a-distance is successful, that the healing is progressing smoothly? Trust and faith questions could also be asked here . . . Why do you do TT? How do you know it is making a difference?

- I experience the success of healing at-a-distance as a feeling of peaceful comfort and connection with the healing partner. I also feel extremely focused.
- Sense of deep peace and harmony in the healing partner's field.
- Impression of the patient as more relaxed or sleeping. Intuitive sense to stop and let him rest.
- More than a relaxation response, I have a "clunk" perception—the psychic equivalent of something snapping into place or of something starting to flow out or fill in—just as I do when I do a treatment in person.
- I see the person as whole and healthy—often stretching and smiling.
- I feel the universal healing energy working through me and going to the healee.
- More like field opens and presents info/communicates. The energy shifts and responds—no sense of being shut out. Can feel energy field change.
- Sense changes in the healing partner's field from my first assessment; I verify these with the healee and family.
- I am only aware of the field and how the energy flow is changing from disorder to order—no physical awareness at all.
- Over time there seems to be a smoothing and greater integration of the whole field with fewer and fewer cues and areas of "pay attention to me." As well, the person will come to mind less and less as needing a treatment.
- I receive many types of visual signals that tell me of the patient's progress and when the person has had enough.
- I note a shift in consciousness, and then complete, as if "done," and hope/pray for the best. Or I may note that my hand chakras have cooled, no longer tingle.
- I don't concern myself with the success; it has its own wisdom. How it appears may be different from the outcome. It is in process.
- If I'm on the phone with the healing partner, by verbal/tonal feedback.

Awareness of Completion of the Treatment

How do you know when the treatment is finished for that session? When the experience has been spaceless and timeless, how does the healer know that the session is "at an end"?

- I sense that the field has cleared and the guiding intelligences confirm.
- In reassessment—hand moves through field with no hovering.
- Sometimes I get reassurance that I've finished.
- There is mutual agreement between our two Inner Selves that we are "done" and there is a shift in color of the healing partner's field—it is more flowing, fuller/brighter color.
- I sense "enough" and then disconnect from the healing partner's field. I'm not sure what precipitates this.
- It feels as if the healing partner and I agree at a subtle level of awareness that it is time to end.
- There is a shift in awareness from out there to local, whether that is in my physical self or my surroundings.
- A sense of symmetry and flow. Sometimes a sort of beatific psychic smile, but without content.
- My mind's screen usually dims; light that filled it during the treatment begins to fade.
- There is a perception that the client needs to rest—a sense that the client has a lot of internal work that needs care.
- My perception is that the energy has been calmed and the healing is there to be accepted or not.
- My visualization of the partner changes; I often perceive it as a color or shading of the area.
- I know that the treatment is done when I sense that the energy is no longer being absorbed by the healing partner.
- This is the same way I feel when an in-person treatment is completed. When my awareness becomes less focused and/or less centered and I feel less present with the healee, I assume that my opportunity for helping has ended.
- I find that I can take a deep breath more easily once his energy

begins to move. This has happened so frequently that I now use it as a gauge of the effect of the treatment. It seems to relate to the connection as well as the movement of energy, release of blocks, and return to the body being able to balance.

Closure of Healing-at-a-Distance Session

Is there anything you routinely do when you know that a healing treatment has been completed?

- I sit with them for a while and let them rest. I continue to send the healing energy of peace, love, and healing as I gently depart in my mind and come back to myself (body) and environment.
- I send goodwill and thanks. I visualize a clear light surrounding the person and flowing easily from the top to the ground.
- I always wish for the highest good and peace for the healing partner.
- There is deep gratitude. I thank Creator for assisting with the work we have done.
- I visualize the healee bathed in and supported by ethereal light as he rests.

A few healers had not been doing anything particular at the end of sessions, but now felt it was a good idea:

- I am now thinking that I should say something to the healing partner, just as I do after a physical (contact) treatment.
- I think it's a good idea and will start doing it (at least) for my own personal growth.

There was a comment on how short the healing sessions seemed to be:

- It is interesting that healing-at-a-distance sessions seem so short (in a linear way) and there is a sense of great depth to the sessions.

Post-Session Verification

How is the condition of the healing partner verified following the completion of the healing session?

Mainly because the recipients are at an actual distance from the healer, there is difficulty in follow-up to an at-a-distance session. Sometimes a healing partner calls, particularly if the healing session has been successful. Some people communicate regularly via phone or email.

- If it is someone I treat regularly, we communicate regularly about the treatment and the partner's response to it. If it's a one-time treatment, a great deal depends on the healing partner getting in touch.
- Our TT group (routinely) receives email back from the healees reporting on their current condition.
- Conversation with the recipient is usually done during the follow-up sessions.
- Since any good that I may do comes from another source, I never wonder how it has turned out. I have heard from others that a change for the better occurred or an outright healing occurred, but still (I don't think) it has anything to do with me.
- Sometimes I check in again at a distance to see whether anything has changed.
- Whenever possible I seek to verify the healing partner's condition after a treatment, either with the healing partner himself or with another person. I always trust that the healing has occurred for the person exactly as it needs to occur.
- Seeing and responding to colors in the healing partner's field is an important aspect to me. Color guides me more during face-to-face TT treatments, but it is definitely a factor during healing-at-a-distance treatments.
- When I first began distance healing I wanted to prove to myself it worked so I partnered with a fellow TT practitioner. I would send her a treatment at a specific time. After the treatment I would record what I felt and send it to her via e-mail. After her rest she would record what she felt and send it to me—and then read what I had sent. The following week we reversed the process. We were amazed at how much we were picking up from each other.
- I have a distance healing e-mail list comprised of more than one hundred TT practitioners. I have received requests for distance TT

for numbers of people over the years. I send the requests out to my e-mail list by bcc. Not everyone will have the time to distance, but even if a handful can participate, I know that those in need will receive healing. I have asked for updates from the person requesting TT for either a friend, family, colleague, or even themselves (all with permission) for periodic updates so my e-mail list will know if they are to continue offering TT, or when the healee is no longer in need. In this regard I have received a lot of positive feedback that "we" are making a difference. In other cases, apart from my e-mail list, I receive personal requests and that person usually gives me great feedback, including being able to feel the TT session, the pain lessened. So I know this works and is very effective.

Some do healing at-a-distance when the recipient is asleep. One healer reported doing a visualization experiment with a friend in which she "visualized the time we wanted the person to receive treatment. It worked, so (thereafter) that's what we did. If a healee is awake when I can do the session, I phone first and arrange for the person to be where he can lie down and sleep after the session."

Working with Others

Are there occasions when you have participated in healing at-a-distance with others simultaneously in the healer role? If so, under what circumstances?

Most of the forty therapists participating in this study practice healing at-a-distance by themselves, and in addition, about half of these healers also work with a group. As with all of the questions, their answers varied.

- In my TT practice group we usually spend about a quarter of the year devoted to healing at-a-distance. We divide into groups and work with specific people, many of whom have been there with us physically for at least one session. We report back to the group any response or feedback from the medical professionals caring for these healees.

- My first experiences of healing at-a-distance with a group happened at Camp Indralaya. Each morning Dora would lead a meditation, a series of statements always ending with "sending thoughts of peace to the world." Prior to the last statement, Dora would invite us to think of someone or some group who was in need of healing. We were instructed to hold that person or persons in our mind and send thoughts/energy of healing. Sometimes Dora would accept names of individuals, and she would call them out. By the time we got to that point in the meditation, Dora had guided and nurtured the group to feel centered and connected. The experiences—having a sense of energetically connecting with a person, to varying degrees, when the name was called—were very real for me. I would sometimes compare notes with others about what we sensed when different names were mentioned, because we often did feel or sense those energies.

- I worked with others during events where we had meditation practice. I have noticed that these occasions are when I am least likely to notice any details about the healing partner.

- I conduct a monthly TT practicum. Usually there are five, up to ten, individuals present. We begin the meeting with a centering exercise and then sit facing each other in a large circle. Often we do healing at-a-distance as a group for part of the afternoon. Someone in the group suggests a person who would welcome our sending healing. They tell us the name and perhaps a sentence or two about the situation. I remind any new members that as we do healing together we are to hold the healing partner in their highest good. The members of the group, at my suggestion, all silently enter meditation, usually with eyes closed. When I notice that most members of the group have opened their eyes and looked up, signaling they are "done," I verbally suggest that we all come back to be fully present in the room. The meditation lasts about five minutes. I ask if anyone wishes to share what they observed during the healing at-a-distance.

    The descriptions of their experiences and approach vary considerably. Some people bring the person to mind and perform TT, even using physical hand gestures, as if they were doing TT in person. One of our participants recounts "videotapes" that she sees in her mind's eye. These are symbolically meaningful to her. For example, she might see fields of daisies amid mountains and streams near a small cabin. From these symbols she may intuit that the person is rather isolated but has strong physical stamina and good healing potential. Another person may not "see" anything but feels energy information that she interprets as related to the healee's physical pain or anxiety.

I often think of the story of the wise blind men examining an elephant and each describing what they feel as they examine the ears or trunk or leg of the animal. Our descriptions of our experience are as different as we are, but they somehow all relate in a helpful way to the person or situation. The group members enjoy these "healings" together and new participants seem to feel reassured that there are many ways to do this process "inside" and at a distance. We have had several powerful follow-up stories from folks who have personal knowledge of the apparent beneficial effect of our group distance TT. One man felt we helped him recover more quickly from surgery than expected. In most cases, however, we do not have specific follow-up information.

Focus of Consciousness

What is your sense of where your consciousness is focused during healing at-a-distance?

- My consciousness is still well connected, but has traveled from my body to focus on the person needing the healing.
- I get an immediate sensation across the bridge of my nose, extending into my cheeks, when I am in a state of consciousness for this work. It is as if this physical sensation tells me I am in the proper state of consciousness to have communication with this other person.
- Initially my awareness is in my frontal lobes. After solid contact with the recipient has been established, the heart and heart chakra

usually become open to contact, but frontal lobes remain as a primary avenue of communication.

- I may feel their pain or comfort in my body for an instant, just as in a physical session.
- I am focused throughout my core, often including the brow chakra as well. Actually I feel as though all chakras are engaged when I'm truly focused.
- It is best to say that I try to remain outside myself, so I am in a different state of consciousness.
- I get several visuals and that seems to occupy my full attention. My consciousness is focused on the healing partner.
- It is through the chakras that I perceive all that I do in these distance sessions.
- I sense that the healing is going successfully because I physically feel the subtle field change.

Conclusions: What We Understand, What We Know

What follows is a brief summary from existing literature about what we know and what we believe about healing at-a-distance.

Healing at-a-Distance Is Universal

Many people from many cultures all over the planet pray, and have done so for all of history. They petition a large, unseen force for help. They ask for some individual to become better, to heal. Culturally the expressions look different but the core activity—that of appealing to an unseen, nonobjective large "something" to assist—is universal.

The Primary Frame of Techniques

How do they do it? In virtually every culture and society, individuals who are engaged in healing move into an altered state of consciousness. Often they are assisted by group experience, music, chanting, powerful intention, and altered breathing. Or quietly, inwardly, one individual may close her eyes and is immediately "in" another frame of perception.

They deliberately set aside the ordinary activities of life, at least briefly, to enter into relationship with some form of a healing energy. Focusing inwardly on the needs of another, intending the good, yields a mysteriously satisfying interior calm and possibly brings new information to the healer.

Core Avenues for Perceiving Information

The information comes in many forms. Some "just know" within an altered state of consciousness. Others "see" visions, colors, or images. Others "hear" words, music, tones, sounds in nature, or deep silence. Many "feel" meaningful sensations in their bodies, such as hands warming, or heartfelt compassionate emotion.

Primary Incentives

Why do they keep doing it? The experience itself is rewarding, uplifting, joyful, purposeful, meaningful, profound, often touching a core place that is deeply satisfying. The experience has lasting impact on the healer and on the object of the healing. The healer becomes more proficient at the process, the longer she practices the activity. The experience of participating in healing practice morphs and increasingly "makes sense" to the healing practitioner, as if another language or way of knowing the world is being learned. Using anecdotal evidence, through self-reflection, the healer concludes that something tangible and important is being accomplished by the process. Faith, initially blind, is bolstered by experiential evidence. Some of these experiences are so deeply meaningful to the healer that the memory of them lasts a lifetime. The act of prayerful healing is repeated over time, thus transforming the healer's life way.

Profiles of at-a-Distance Healers

Who are these healers? Do those drawn to healing inhabit a subset of psychic profiles? The Minnesota Multiphasic Personality Inventory (MMPI), a standardized psychological test of adult personality and psychopathology, was administered to a group of Therapeutic Touch healers. Analysis of the data concluded that the subjects were "remarkable for their normality," although heterogeneous in individual patterns.* Are some more sensitive to psychic experiences and therefore drawn to practice them? Conversely, among those sensitives, some may choose to avoid those experiences.

Similarity to Intercessory Prayer

Healing with Therapeutic Touch is close to blessing the healing partner. For some, healing at-a-distance is similar and perhaps interchangeable with intercessory prayer. This form of prayer is understood by many Christians as a request for intervention, one of the five major types of prayer. Other forms of Christian prayer are prayer of adoration, in praise of the greatness of God, prayer of contrition or acknowledgment of sinfulness, prayer of love or charity, and prayer of thanksgiving.

Healers have a very strong belief in the "rightness" of what they are doing. The experience of healing at-a-distance can occur at such psychological depth that the healer is often unable to adequately verbalize the experience. She may describe deeply personal and profound experiences, even to herself, in very simple language that belies the full depth of meaning. TT healers may have profound experiences through sentience that are essentially difficult or impossible to be translated into words.

What Do They Not Experience?

No one has any trouble "coming back" to ordinary perception. No one describes any untoward personal consequences from these practices. They do not describe feeling worse, physically or emotionally, after their healing-at-a-distance experience. This is in contrast to descriptions in some cultures of the shaman taking on the illness of the client, thus resulting in impaired personal physical health.† Nearly universally healers indicate they feel better, even felt "healed" themselves, after the healing-at-a-distance experience.

No one describes the client feeling worse after the at-a-distance

---

*C. Brown, R. Fischer, A. Wagman, N. Horrom, P. Marks, "The EEG in Meditation and Therapeutic Touch Healing," *Journal of Altered States of Consciousness* 3 (1978): 169–80.
†K. C. Krycka, "Shamanic Practices and the Treatment of Life-Threatening Medical Conditions," *Journal of Transpersonal Psychology* 32 (2000): 69–88.

healing experience on his behalf. Many in fact invite additional healing for themselves, sensing that it is somehow helpful. Some people who are especially sensitive may prefer not to be "prayed on," perhaps out of a sense of potential overwhelm or protection of personal privacy.

The healers describe increasing confidence in their effectiveness and increasing meaning as they perform these healings at a distance over time, some over many years. No one in this study indicated wariness or warnings about potential psychic dangers. This may be a testament to the essential psychic hardiness of this group, or naïveté, or a function of the convenience sample by which they were asked to self-select to participate.

It must be noted that, upon reflection, the authors of the study came to realize that none of the TT therapists were asked directly about negative experiences related to healing at-a-distance. Thus there is a follow-up summary in answer to the question of what happens when things don't go as planned.

Major Limitations of the Study

As noted, the size of the study sample was forty Therapeutic Touch therapists, each of whom had at least three years of experience with TT. It was an exploratory study and not meant to attain statistical reliability; however, a larger, more defined sample would add to its credibility. The descriptions of experience are likely to be familiar to other modern groups, such as Christian prayer ministries or cloistered religious communities.

The age of this study group was roughly late 40s to 90s. Virtually all had been practicing TT for more than five years, and many for more than twenty. There were no children, adolescents, or even young adults in the demographics of this group. All participants were of European descent residing in the United States or Canada. All but two respondents in this study were female.

Major Findings of the Study

What did we learn from this healing-at-a-distance study? Despite their idiosyncratic descriptions of altered states of consciousness, there is an underlying coherence among these Therapeutic Touch practitioners. These modern TT practitioners, including laypersons as well as many who work in clinical helping professions such as nursing, teaching, and other related healthcare professions, readily enter a world of phenomena that would be familiar to ancient shamans and mystics.

Many framed their healing style on Therapeutic Touch principles and approached the process as they might if the healing partner were physically present. They described recurrent rhythms such as specific colors or patterns "seen," "sounds heard," or sometimes feeling within a wave of enveloping silence. They recounted "feeling" changes in their bodies (for example, hands get "warm and tingling") reminiscent of their in-person TT healing experiences.

Almost universally they described feeling a joyful "upliftment" from the radiant "light" they "saw," and a humble sense of gratitude for the privilege of entering this healing encounter. They described experiencing peace, love, wholeness, timelessness, and unity, as well as openness. Many described sensing that they were assisted by nonphysical beings. They recognized these beings as familiar, loving, and helpful. Sometimes they discerned that the "loving energy" was already connected to the healee, and sometimes it occurred when the healer invited the help.

They described entering or traveling in an altered state of consciousness. Variously they were in touch with their physical surroundings and personal bodies. Some "left" their bodies, feeling themselves to be entirely in spirit form in order to encounter the other. They described being permeated by the energy or rhythm of the healee. Some reported that they could "see" inside the physical body or "sense" emotional turmoil that often gradually smoothed or subsided as they worked with the person.

The TT practitioners described entering a profound stillness or "sea of silence" during healing at-a-distance. Some could "hear" sounds or tones, occasionally words or music. Some "received" messages that guided their practice or "knowings" to be conveyed to the healee. They described "feeling" the messages or "hearing them in my head," rather than hearing them with their physical ears. They also described mind-to-mind communication with the healee.

9

Healing-at-a-Distance Case Studies

The following studies detail experiences of trained therapists who agreed to participate in research into the process of Therapeutic Touch healing at-a-distance. In other words, none of them were in the same physical location as their healing partners.

Case 1

Sleep and Healing

A therapist finds that sleep during or after a distance session potentiates the healing.

In the Beginning

The treatment begins as soon as I have the thought that I will give my healing partner a treatment. As I get myself physically comfortable, I am already becoming centered. I take a deep breath and begin by trying to visualize my healing partner. Sometimes I am successful, but as soon as my hands begin to move, the visualization disappears and I find that I am working with the pulsing of the field.

I always begin with something that looks very much like the TT learned in my basic level; this is my ritual that takes me deeper to sustained centering, in touch with my Inner Self. At some point in the treatment I begin to use my hand or hands to move down the field. I don't see a field; I sense the "localization" that is the healing partner's field. The hands hover at points where there are imbalances or congestion, until the field is brought to order at that point. If the hovering seems to be taking a long time, I often unruffle the area and then start over with my hands moving down the field.

Perception of Self

I do distance TT in two ways. Most of the time I am upstairs in a chair and I am "beside" the healing partner, but only my upper chakras are there with my hands. I'm aware of my hands moving, but only sense the palm and fingertip chakras; it is as if those are the only parts of me that exist in the "other place" of my consciousness. The lower chakras keep me grounded in my space-time body. I am conscious of them humming along in the background, but they are not involved in the treatment.

Sometimes I am in bed and do my TT just before I go to sleep. In this case I am doing it all as a visualization—still aware of my hands moving through the field, even though they are not moving as I lie in my bed. In this case I feel as though I am "out there" as a presence working in a field of awareness. This is extremely difficult to explain.

Sounds Heard

Sometimes an imbalance sounds to me like an orchestra tuning up—a real cacophony. Then, as I work to rebalance, the orchestra starts to play a Strauss waltz and I know that things are smoothing out.

I hear voices from time to time. Sometimes they make me aware of the emotions felt by my healing partner and the reason for the way he is feeling. Sometimes I'm told to hover a bit longer—to be patient (something I am working on in this lifetime). Other times I hear encouragement if I think I'm not feeling anything.

Memory

Sometimes before sleeping I feel a pulsing, like I am part of an ocean of energy; colors are golden/red and I get the feeling that I am deeply centered—at one with my Inner Self and with the healing partner. When I connect deeply to my Inner Self it is as though he is my most beloved friend; my heart throbs and I feel a deep love and sense of gratitude and a longing to be closer.

Perception of the Ambience

If I know where the healing partner is, I'll have a glimpse of his environment when I visualize him at the start of the session, but that fades when I start into the treatment. I am aware of angelic presences or family members who have passed on, most often when working with someone close to death.

Mind-to-Mind Communication

I feel I am in mind-to-mind communication with the healee; I sometimes talk to him in my mind and get the feeling that I am heard. I don't get answers, just feeling. Sometimes words well up from my heart chakra, and I feel the connection heart-to-heart.

Awareness of a Presence

I feel the sense of the healee's field, connecting heart-to-heart. Sometimes there is a very deep connection with my Inner Self. I can feel connected to my guide and angel, and to a team of ascended masters on the other side.

Success of Treatment

I have a sense of the field and how the flow of the energy is changing from disorder to order.

Awareness of Completion of the Treatment

In reassessment, my hand moves through the field with no hovering.

Closure of Treatment

I nearly always end with a Christian benediction—a remnant from my upbringing.

Post-Session Verification

I usually do my distance TT at a time when I know the person will be asleep and stay sleeping until morning. I did a yearlong study with a friend, another Recognized Teacher, sharing distance TT. We tried all sorts of things. We found that if we visualized a clock at the start of our treatment, and set it to when we wanted our healee to receive the treatment, it worked. So that's what I do now. If I do distance TT during a time when the person might be awake, I phone first and arrange for him to be in a place where he can sleep after the session.

Focus of Consciousness

At the start my consciousness is heart-to-heart communication through the heart chakra, as well as throat, third eye, and crown chakras. My hand and fingertip chakras are also involved, communicating with my upper chakras. And I am connected to my Inner Self, sometimes very deeply.

Case 2

Light, Easy, and Elegant

A therapist finds that although measurement of a treatment in linear time might be four to six minutes these distance sessions can have great depth.

In the Beginning

I take a deep abdominal breath and close my eyes. When I first began doing distance healing I used a photo of the person and kept my eyes open. Now I close my eyes and focus my attention and intention on the person with whom I am doing the healing work. It is absolutely essential for my physical body to be comfortable.

I engage in all dimensions of centering including relaxing my body, allowing my mind to become quiet, focusing my attention on the recipient, setting my intention for the recipient's highest good, opening my awareness to whatever information the field offers me, allowing myself to be a conduit for healing energy, and asking what needs to be done.

The centering brings me more directly in communication with my

Inner Self. It is as if "I" am the observer and "someone else" is the driver of the process; it is all so easy and elegant.

I listen deeply with my entire being: seeing, hearing, feeling (emotion and sensory), smelling, tasting—all senses are involved and are on high alert.

Do I visualize the healing partner? It depends on each experience. There are times when I have a clear image of the physical body of the healing partner. Sometimes there is only a sense of the energetic field as a whole; and at other times there is a sense only of aspects of the field that require attention in the specific moment.

There is a sense of deep connection with the healing partner and a clear sense that he is receptive to the process and the healing energy that is about to be sent. There is a readiness to begin on the part of the recipient as well as on my part; sometimes the centering and the readiness are instantaneous. There have been occasions when I have sat down to do a healing session with a specific person and it has been as if the "screen is blank," there is no one home. I have come to recognize and realize that this is not the right time for this person to receive healing energy. On several occasions I have actually heard the words "no one is home," and now recognize that it is not the time to do healing with that person. When this first happened I questioned myself—was I doing something wrong? However, it became clear to me that this was about the healing partner and that person's needs and desires, not about me at all.

Perception of Self

I don't really "see" myself; it is an inner feeling, or felt sense. There are times when I feel in a meditative state and energy is moving through and from me to the healing partner. Other times it is as if my physical being is pure energy so there is no "me" sitting on the chair in this location; my energy meets the energy of the recipient somewhere (the location is not defined) and we interact with each other.

When I first did distance healing I imagined myself with the partner and physically doing TT as if I were physically present with him. Now my physical being is not visible where our energies are interacting.

Occasionally I am aware of sensations and images being localized in my head, but this is not always the experience. Often the information and energy exchange is undefined in terms of location.

I don't typically see myself with other beings. However, I have occasionally had a sense of other beings supporting the process, and there are times when I feel drawn to asking for the healee's angels and supportive beings to assist with the process. There is a sense of the process being enhanced by these supportive beings.

It is clear that my conscious mind is not doing anything within the interaction; I am the observer of the process that is leading and giving what needs to be done. My role is one of witnessing the process and noting what has happened so that this information can be recorded and relayed to the healee, if needed.

Sense of Place

The light is a physical sense of lightness, airiness, spaciousness, expansiveness, as if the molecules in my physical being are separated by huge spaces; I am so light that I could float like a helium balloon.

I would say that the atmosphere is one of certainty; certainty that what needs to be done in this moment will indeed be done. There is quiet anticipation, a soft excitement and eagerness.

Sometimes there are swooshing sounds that I would attribute to moving energy rather than wind. I sense movement of energy that flows like water; however, I haven't thought of it as moving waters.

There is a deep quiet that feels as though I am basking in that silence. As I think about it now, it is as if within the quiet "all is perceived." There is no effort; the information comes quickly and easily.

In that place where the interaction occurs is a deep sense of peacefulness and quietude. The stillness and quietude are profound, and there is a deep sense of connecting with the recipient. There is a deep sense of knowing that there is no separation; we are one—what the other feels, I feel, and as the other experiences healing, I also heal. It is a profound experience, one that I feel very honored to share with the healee.

Olfactory Sensations

There are times when I have experienced something that could be termed a smell; however, it does not seem important to label the experience as an aroma—it just is.

Sounds Heard

I hear words regularly; other sounds, infrequently. When energy that is blocked begins to move I sometimes hear a sound and see an image as if a log jam has just opened up and the river is flowing. Occasionally I feel the flowing sensation in my body.

Memory

I have memories of feeling energy opening, flowing, or releasing in my body. Sometimes a session can feel like déjà vu even if I do not consciously remember a specific experience.

Mind-to-Mind Communication

I don't feel mind-to-mind communication with the healee but rather with my own Inner Self. It is as if my inner wisdom is guiding the entire process. I trust the process that takes place, and begin the interaction when I center and set the intention. There is a wisdom that infuses the entire process; I just open myself to that wisdom. It is as if I am in an ocean of knowingness that guides the process, and I am plugged in to this knowingness.

Awareness of a Presence

Very specific information comes when I focus on the recipient. This can be patterns of energy flow—colors, characteristics of the energy imbalances (for example, heavy, thick, gray)—in images or colors. The entire process is guided by a greater wisdom. There is a sense of knowing that permeates the experience. I know that what happens during the session is for the highest good and the greater good of the healee. I know that I can and do trust the process.

Success of Treatment

How I sense this: The field shifts and changes until the session is complete. I get a sense that something more needs to be done and my attention opens to what that is—and then it happens. Sometimes it just happens without my being aware that something more needs to be done. There is an intelligence in the healee's energy field that guides the process to successful completion. I bear witness to the process from a privileged position.

Awareness of Completion of the Treatment

The change in the communication with my Inner Self is as if the connection is no longer there, as if someone turned off the screen where everything was happening. When the session is complete, the energy stops shifting and changing. Sometimes there is a sound, like a "clunk," as if the pieces have fit together in the way they need to connect. Other times I hear *done,* and there is a clear sense that the session is finished.

Closure of Treatment

Sometimes I say thank you for the privilege of working with the healee. Sometimes there is an abrupt end and the channel of communication is severed; there is a sense of ending. Occasionally I have heard the words "rest, relax, peace."

I have been recording the sessions for several years. It is challenging to capture all the nuances of the experience because a session happens so quickly. The sessions are four to six minutes. It is interesting that the distance healing sessions are so short in linear time, and there is a sense of great depth.

Post-Session Verification

I do not typically ask the healee later how he feels. Many of the people on our healing request list are those whom I have never met, and they are at considerable distance from me. There is a sense at the end of the session that what needed to be done at that moment in time has been done.

Afterwards our group occasionally receives an e-mail from the recipient of a family member to indicate that the person is feeling better or has died.

Much of the information I receive during the TT session and at the end is visual. I receive a lot of color information, pattern information; and I sometimes experience sensations in my physical body of heaviness, lightness, release, flowing. I see changes in clarity of the energy: muddiness to clarity; heaviness to lightness; red to pink, then blue or green; heavy, swirling motions to softer flowing, and more even flowing. Sometimes I feel a difference in sensations in my physical body—a heaviness on one side, or on one side of my head. These physical sensations are brief, as if they are providing me with additional information with which to understand the healee's experience and to make sense out of what is happening. It is as if this information is to help my conscious mind understand what I am observing.

Focus of Consciousness

My heart feels open but I would say that my entire being is open and receptive. I am sometimes aware of energy from my solar plexus. My consciousness does not recognize parts; it feels like a whole. My consciousness is focused with my intention. My focus feels narrow and expansive at the same time.

Case 3

Center of Center

A therapist feels that during the process her consciousness shifts into a different dimension that is like being inside the universe where there is no separation of time and space.

In the Beginning

I take a deep breath and center. I get in touch with my Inner Self, listen deeply, and visualize the healing partner. I relax into my heart chakra and come into conscious harmony with that universal healing energy.

Perception of Self

I am aware of where I am physically but I have also connected in another time dimension with the healee, so I am with him, too. My consciousness is present with the person, and at the same time I am in a different time dimension, like the inside of the universe where there is no separation of time and space; I'm consciously present there.

Sense of Place
I feel an atmosphere of silence, and it feels like I am inside the universe where time and space are different from the way they are on Earth. It is very quiet. Like the center of center.

Memory
This is unique for me—this experience. I don't remember ever experiencing anything like it before. It is distinct unto itself.

Perception of the Ambience
Sometimes I am aware of the environment of the healing partner and energetic allies. I mostly am aware of whether the person is sleeping or active, and what kind of sleep it is (peaceful or agitated). I can sense if the partner is distracted. I think I pick up on his emotional state.

Mind-to-Mind Communication
My experience of mind-to-mind communication is between the healing partner and my Inner Self.

Awareness of a Presence
I feel the presence of that profound quiet of the inner workings of the universe. (Seems so funny to write that, as if I know what the inner workings of the universe feel like, but that's the only way I can describe it right now in my current state of understanding.) It feels as if I am in the experience of harmony with the universe and its laws of nature/life.

Awareness of Completion of the Treatment
My Inner Self informs me of the change when the treatment is complete.

Closure of Treatment
I have done some experiments with other TT people to learn distance TT and we usually compare notes afterward. It's very educational to

learn from others how they perceive the closure of treatments at a distance.

Post-Session Verification

Sometimes I ask the healee how he feels, but I may also rely on my own sense of the situation.

Focus of Consciousness

I am aware of being in unity with the universal healing energy.

Case 4

Healing at-a-Distance at the End of Life

A therapist is able to assist the dying process from a hundred miles away.

I have had a number of experiences in distance healing, but one in particular was significant because it involved a witness.

My husband G was dying at home. One day my daughter L and her husband were visiting. We were sitting in the next room when I heard the Cheyne-Stokes respirations begin. (This is a change in breathing pattern that can be very noisy and often indicates imminent death. It can be very disturbing to loved ones.) I said, "It's time for Therapeutic Touch!"

L came with me and as I did TT, witnessed the calming effects until my husband's breathing returned to normal. Then she and her husband went out for a walk, and while they were gone, G died in my arms and I "saw the light" as his "essence" moved into it.

The following year J, the father of L's husband, was in the hospital (about 100 miles away) and death was expected to be soon. At 7:30 p.m. L phoned me in tears, saying, "J has that awful breathing! Even the nurses are upset. Can you do something?" I assured her I would try. So I centered and pictured J in my mind. I did the moves that I sensed were required for perhaps two to three minutes.

At 7:40 p.m. the phone rang and L was again sobbing—but with relief. She said, "Mom, you're awesome!"

J rested peacefully during the night.

The next morning I woke unexpectedly at 7 o'clock and sat quietly. At 7:10 a.m. J "appeared" in front of me, looking confused. I said to him, "It's time to leave—go to the light." He looked around and said, "Well, there's an awful lot of it!" And with that he turned and gradually faded from sight into a white mist.

I phoned L who confirmed that his death had been recorded as 7:12 a.m. She said, "I knew you would know."

Case 5

Light, Love, Bliss

A therapist experiences heart-to-heart communication with the healee.

In the Beginning
- I start by asking to serve as an instrument of healing.
- I seek what is the highest and best for the healee.
- I scan my field to identify my own emotions and breathe deeply to release any personal outcome desires.

Perception of Self
I am aware of heart-center and third-eye activation.

Sense of Place
It is a transcendent place without three-dimensional reference.

Sounds Heard
The "sights" and "sounds" I experience are not within the realm of the five senses. These words are the best metaphors for my perceptions. Occasionally a "voice" provides a message for a loved one. Sometimes there is succinct information to be conveyed to the healee—always in a constructive, supportive, and loving tone.

Memory
Sometimes visualizations spontaneously occur of an imaginative aspect, which culminate in unity of a transcendent nature with the healee.

When it has been described to the person, the content has been reported to have resonance for him.

Perception of the Ambience
Generally distance healing has the nonspecific ambience of "open-ended silence," but specifics are visible if they serve as confirmation or validation of the healing process.

Mind-to-Mind Communication
I would say communication is more heart-to-heart than mind-to-mind. The connection can be intense and discernible.

Success of Treatment
There is a sense of deep peace and harmony.

Awareness of Completion of the Treatment
Frequently when the treatment is complete I "see" an inner blue light at my third eye. Conversely, if I inadvertently end a healing before completion I sense a magnetic force holding me in place to continue further.

Post-Session Incident Verification
While it is not my routine practice to communicate about each healing with the healee, I generally stay in touch with the spouse and the family—if appropriate—to let them know I'm working with the person daily. If a distance healing is especially strong, or if information comes through intended for the healee, of course I convey the information. Responses have affirmed benefit.

Working with Others
I conduct healing at-a-distance daily by myself, and I sometimes attend a meditation group where it is practiced. I annually attend five-day retreats where distance healing is taught and practiced.

Focus of Consciousness
The healing connection seems to emanate from the heart chakra in alignment with the crown and pineal centers, but the most profound

healings seem to transcend physical awareness in a realm of light, love, and bliss.

Case 6

Connection and Communication
at a Distance

A therapist finds that perceiving changes in the healee's field feels similar to in-person sessions.

In the Beginning

I start by accepting the gender, first name, and geographic location of the client into my consciousness. I relax physically, then mentally; I feel for the "meld" with my Inner Self. At this point the personal shift/connection is with what I consider to be my spirit self, rather than with the deeper aspect of my soul.

Perception of Self

This part of treatment is always the same. My physical and Inner Self awareness operate smoothly as one unit. I/we combine our joined awareness and focus on the general geographic location, then open up the search capability to locate the entity matching the known description, including issues when that has been part of the description. Feeling (mental not physical) for a connection between the healee and the person who asked me to help this individual is a further check that I have located the right person. I then gently approach the healee in my consciousness, introduce myself, explain why I'm there, and explain the general procedure. I make sure the healee understands and is in charge, can accept or reject my offer to assist, and can stop the session at any time if desired. As in an in-person healing, this session is between the healee and me only.

Sense of Place

My preference is to be in and aware of the physical location of the healee. As often as not, during the locating of the healee my focus is tightly controlled on him to the exclusion of the setting. As that is happening we seem to be surrounded by a thin white fog that is without sensation.

Sounds Heard

Occasionally there may be a mild rushing sound during the initial locating of the healee. During the session it is common to "hear" bodily functions of the healee.

Mind-to-Mind Communication

Most often, the session is limited to the client's physical body. Sometimes the Inner Self of the person is involved.

Awareness of a Presence

The other presences are higher aspects of the healee and of me. I don't recall ever being aware of spiritual presences during a session.

Success of Treatment

As happens during an in-person healing, I may see or sense a change in the body or aura of the healee. I may sense glow, temperature change, sounds, or movement, or become aware of lessening of discomfort.

Awareness of Completion of the Treatment

I have a sense of satisfaction that brings the realization it is time to stop. The healee may seem fully relaxed and sleepy to me. Also, there is a slight but growing awareness of my physical body.

Closure of Treatment

I talk mind-to-mind to the client as I would if it were not a distance session.

Post-Session Verification

Usually a follow-up treatment is in order. Then I may have a conversation with the healee to hear his personal evaluation.

Focus of Consciousness

Initially my consciousness is in my frontal lobes. After solid contact has been established, my heart and heart chakra usually become open to contact, but the frontal lobes remain the primary avenue.

<u>Case 7</u>

Communicating with the Extended Mind

A therapist experiences knowing things that "I do not know how I know."

In the Beginning

I get physically comfortable, take a deep breath, and close my eyes. I center my consciousness. I get in touch with my Inner Self and allow myself to sink into another place in my mind's eye and in my body. I listen deeply. I attempt to visualize the healing partner, but this often does not occur; the visions come in colors and shapes that seem unique to the individual and change over time, and perhaps change during the course of the healing session. The visions occur fairly quickly in the process, usually within the first few seconds.

Perception of Self

Usually I experience myself quietly meditating in my meditation chair. Sometimes I can see myself applying TT with my hand chakras to the healee, as if I am at the bedside. Sometimes the person appears as if before me, or a part of him, such as heart chakra swirls, may appear. I am most aware of my mind's eye and heart-torso area. Often my hands tingle. Other beings are instantly available when I call upon them; usually they speak in my mind. They are very familiar presences, loving and helpful.

Sense of Place

The atmosphere is very peaceful; lights, shapes, and colors are always present. It is a lovely "place" to be and I feel uplifted as I return to ordinary life. I do not hear music or instruments, birds or the wind, or moving waters. It is very quiet. It is difficult to distinguish what I am perceiving. Sometimes the patterns or colors suggest symbolically something I can make sense of cognitively, but often they do not. This place is wordless, silent, calm, and softly enveloping.

Memory

The calm, peaceful feeling is one I associate with lovely spiritual experiences or meditations I have had.

Perception of the Ambience

I do sometimes perceive the environment of the healing partner, including furniture in the room. I don't feel other people in the room but I do sometimes sense energetic allies.

Mind-to-Mind Communication

I feel that I am in communication not so much with the partner's conscious mind but with his extended mind. I feel in communication with my own Inner Self. Sometimes I know things that I do not know how I know. I assume that the energetic intelligences are in communion with my Inner Self. I am not directly aware of that communion.

Success of Treatment

I note a shift in my consciousness and then complete as if done, and hope and pray for the best. Or I may note that my hand chakras have cooled and no longer tingle.

Awareness of Completion of the Treatment

I sometimes feel a change in the healee. I notice that I have returned to my ordinary consciousness and have left his realm.

Post-Session Verification

I usually rely on my own sense of the outcome. Often I do not know the patient personally and so have no contact. Sometimes I get feedback from family or the person directly.

Focus of Consciousness

My focus is typically in my heart and heart chakra, in my hand chakras, and in my mind's eye.

Three Stories of Receiving Healing at-a-Distance

These stories were included in the responses from three of the therapists who were on the receiving end of healing at-a-distance at a time when they were dealing with serious illness. Each of these accounts eloquently describes the reality that TT can help even when symptoms continue.

Strength, Courage, and an Incredible Peace

Several years ago I received distance healing in a deeply profound way from the hearts of healers. And it started with K. I was lying in my bed, burning up with fever and experiencing an intense headache. This had come on acutely during the afternoon as my husband S and I were at the theatre with our family. I could feel myself getting sicker and sicker, and by the time I arrived home I was a goner. S was pretty freaked, and so was I. The phone rang; it was K. I did not know that it was she calling, but I could sense something happening to me in that moment; I would call it seeking of ease—somehow a deep inner peace that did not make my temp drop or my head stop aching but did bring a calm, and core strength to be with those feelings. I really did not know what was happening; I felt like I was literally transitioning yet I was so calm. "Yay for meditation," I thought. S came upstairs and told me that K had called because she sensed there was something very wrong, and she told him it was my right lung. Interestingly, my breath was easy. Later that night, as I became more febrile, I went to the emergency room. Long story short—several X-rays and a CT later—the diagnosis was revealed: pronounced right whole-lung pneumonia.

As I recovered, each day, at different times, I could feel—as a whole-being sense—the presence of others supporting me, somehow giving me strength, courage, and an incredible peace to live with this very long and arduous healing. I knew I was not alone, and I was clear when others connected with me energetically. With K, I could actually see her in person, and we did confirm the experiences. With the others, sometimes I thought I might know who was with me and sometimes I just felt a presence.

A Deep Peace Connection

As a recipient of healing energy when I was so ill in the ER last year, with people dashing around me, I was aware the minute energy was being sent and felt surrounded by a wonderful calming, very gentle blue energy that seemed to penetrate my being. There was a deep knowing that I was "held" and everything would be fine. No matter the outcome, all would be well. It brought peace, tolerance, awareness, and an ability to be "with" what was happening, to go through it and not be swallowed up by fear. There were multiple occasions when this exact scenario played out—a downturn in my health prompted distance TT followed by stabilization with a deep peace connection and knowing I would be okay.

My three children have benefitted from TT—each one in a profound way—and now I have too; I believe it saved my life. TT and my wonderful healing partners held me in balance until the medical profession could catch up with what had actually happened, correct their diagnoses, and stop their life-threatening treatments. I am forever grateful and thank Dee from the bottom of my heart for her gift of Therapeutic Touch.

Healing at-a-Distance Transcends Time and Mortality

I met Dora Kunz in fall of 1974, having just been diagnosed with a rare blood cancer. Life expectancy was ten years. Dora invited me to attend a Pumpkin Hollow Farm Therapeutic Touch Invitational in 1975. For four years she gave me five days of daily twenty-minute treatments during the weeklong TT workshops at Pumpkin Hollow. This was augmented by weekly TT practitioner sessions and meditative self-healing during the rest of the year. TT and meditation were my only healing interventions, since my hematologist offered no allopathic medicine. Forty-seven years later I'm still in remission. My husband and I became friends with Dora. She symbolizes for me healing consciousness.

With deep appreciation for the healing I received, I learned the practice of Therapeutic Touch with Dora and Dee Krieger during thirty-five years at Pumpkin Hollow Farm Invitationals. Distance healing for others and self-healing (meditative, heart-centered awareness to serve as a channel of healing intent) are now a daily practice.

I learned through personal experience that "presence" is definitely perceived in distance healing. In the midst of a heart attack on October 5, 2007, I had a near-death experience on the operating table. I survived the operation with one stent inserted, but with the left anterior descending artery 100 percent occluded; the doctors, in their haste to revive me, had failed to open essential subsidiary arteries. I had a second heart attack five days later with a second stent positioned.

Post-operatively recovering at home, in the midst of self-healing I called upon Dora, who distinctly appeared at the foot of my bed. She had died eight years earlier, in August 1999. As I lay there, heart-connected with Dora, a powerful energy wave passed over my body, pinning my head to the pillow. I felt light throughout my body, and warmth. When the energy dissipated I was profoundly peaceful and my entire body tingled. I felt enormous gratitude. Dora's healing peace and presence remained with me during recovery.

10

Healing-at-a-Distance Challenges and Considerations

While we were involved in this in-depth analysis, we realized we had inadvertently missed an opportunity to be more fully holistic in our core perceptions of this healing act. Nowhere in the study questionnaire had we given responders a prompt that other than positive responses were invited; for instance, any unexpected occurrences that may have happened to the healer, the healing partner, or within the healing situation or environment that had negative effects on either the healer, the healing partner, or the healing process. We asked the study's respondents to help us through this dilemma. We sent out a request to the participants, with some suggestions of ways the distance healing sessions may have in some way been less than successful. It was hypothesized that a negative result might occur in healing at-a-distance for these possible reasons:

- Healers with strong emotions may not realize the overwhelming effect they can have when they inadvertently focus those emotional loads toward healing partners.
- The healer may become overcome by the psychodynamic effects of grief displayed as thought forms surrounding the healee, carried by relatives or friends of the recipient.

- The healer, through lack of experience or understanding of the dynamic effects of subtle energies, may inadvertently leave her personal vital-energy and psychodynamic fields open, unprotected, and therefore vulnerable.
- The healer may have failed to adequately ground herself.
- The healer may be inappropriately ego-focused.
- If there is a close emotional relationship between the healer and healee, the healer may be unable to enter an impersonal space because she is not fully grounded and centered.

Responses to Unexpected Considerations

Out of the original 268 responses, ten people reported negative incidents during healing-at-a-distance events:

- The healer failed to sufficiently ground or center herself.
- The healer was overcome by the grief of the recipient's relatives or friends.
- The offer of doing healing at-a-distance was refused.
- People present in the room had negative attitudes.
- There was a lack of positive relationship with the client.
- The healer expended too much energy and had consequent headache or nausea.

There were no lasting effects of any of the reportedly mild physical symptoms, which included headache, nausea, and some muscular discomfort, all of brief duration.

A close examination of the difficulties provides support for the emphasis on sustained centering. If a therapist begins to feel the feelings of the healee, or if she "expends too much energy," she will learn a lesson about her centering practice that nothing else can so clearly teach. Some healers are naturally highly sensitive; it is the responsibility of each person to know herself and maintain the centered state during Therapeutic Touch, whether in-person or at a distance. Participants reported that it was the healer who experienced discomfort in these instances. Our relatively small study (and many others focusing on healing and prayer) speaks to the reality of the transpersonal energetic interaction—even across miles. The data here supports much anecdotal experience that in most cases healing at-a-distance goes well.

Editor's Note: Reporting from the Laboratory of the Self

As we read over the responses from these TT therapists who are looking honestly at some of the healing-at-a-distance sessions that may not have gone so well, we were reminded of the charge by Dora and Dee to test everything out in the Laboratory of the Self. These therapists are honestly reporting from those laboratories.

Acknowledging an Off Day

On occasion, when I [as healer] am inadequately grounded or too deeply emotionally connected to the healee, I may experience within myself a certain quality of agitation or inappropriate investment in the outcome.

Since I do distance healing daily with people who I know are also often receiving healing from others, I have not confirmed whether the healee has experienced my sense of agitation; there are too many variables to make this determination with validity. I just compassionately—from as neutral a perspective as possible—recognize that this is an off day.

Reaffirming the Importance of Grounding and Centering

I have experienced discomfort in giving TT when not sufficiently grounded. It can feel like being bombarded with sensations. I can feel disconnected from my own self and vulnerable to other psychic energy. By this I mean that I'm not sure whose "stuff" I'm picking up, mine or someone else's.

A lack of centering also can occur—my mind interferes, I get distracted and have to re-center. This can make me frustrated and impatient—my stuff! I can become judgmental toward myself, which makes me question what is "real." Am I nuts? If I don't understand the information/context of the impressions, I feel somewhat confused. It's like I cannot interpret the images—like being in a dream.

I have a hard time distinguishing a "treatment" from placing the partner in the universal healing field—meaning, to me, sending a prayer for his greatest good. My distance TT sessions often have this quality to them, and then I often find myself thinking of the person at a later date and sending more *good* thoughts/energy. I wonder if perhaps I have not really ended the treatment and feel unduly connected or attached.

I can have the sense that I am a voyeur, that even though the person requests distance TT, he is not responsive or open. It's like having a door shut on you—keep out! So I do.

On the positive side I think that distance TT can bring me more intimately to the emotional and mental/spiritual fields. This can be more of a connection than working on a body. I tend to work hands off, so I feel very comfortable in this type of healing environment. I see it as an environment that I am creating. It brings me to a sense of oneness more easily. I feel at ease and less like I'm performing or doing something *to* the healing partner. It is a sense of being with the other.

Relative Accepts In-Person Treatments but Rejects Distance

I have experienced none of the mentioned pitfalls, perhaps due to additional precautions not usually necessary during in-person work.

Probably the closest I've come to a disturbing situation was when I attempted distance work with a niece (who was like a daughter) who was in clinical trials for a glioblastoma. She was aware that the prognosis was terminal. I attempted connection three times and each offer was met with a firm thanks for the offer, but no thank you. Gentle in-person conversations found her keeping things superficial with a hint of evasiveness about her wishes. I did a few in-person treatments with the intention of reducing discomfort and anxiety and left it at that.

Staying Centered When Engaging with Family Members

On occasion I've realized that I am not adequately grounded, but then recognized this and grounded and re-centered.

It's an interesting idea about being off-center because of being emotionally connected with the healee. I sometimes find this when I'm offering TT "hands on" with my children or spouse, so I would ask another practitioner to help out if I'm too close to the situation, especially if it is critical. It's also possible I can really focus on keeping centered so I don't become attached to an outcome. This may have happened occasionally when doing distance healing for my children.

Involving Computers in a Distance Session

I had received an email from a young girl (early twenties) expressing an illness, so I offered distance TT and she accepted; all written communication via emails. So I pushed my chair back from my computer and began to do distance TT. She responded days later that it was an interesting experience to receive the energy, coming out of her computer. That was not my intent of how I was sending the TT but that was her perception of how she received the energy.

Feeling Frozen with Fear of Making a Mistake

I have rarely experienced that one of my Achilles heels gets energetically pricked during a TT session. Thankfully, I can think of this having happened only twice. Growing up, I was severely punished for making even small mistakes, and so a few times I've frozen when I've been afraid that I was going to make a mistake. Both times have been with people who were in much distress. One of the times I stepped out of the field and re-grounded, and then ended the treatment soon after. That was appropriate since that person was quite ill, and I thankfully have not had that reaction since, as I have continued to treat him.

The other thing I know about myself is that I can work too intensely. I come from a culture where some people so thoroughly clean their houses that they also scrub their stoops. I've had to work hard to internalize that I can get the same result and better with less but more-grounded effort. I make a conscious but nonverbal effort to include this realization in my grounding.

Both Therapist and Healee Sense a Disruptive Energy

I was involved in a study with another TT therapist to learn distance TT. I did a distance treatment on her every Tuesday morning at 9 a.m. for about six months. This person was on a remote island and we would have to wait until two days later to do a call to check-in on the treatment.

This particular morning was about three to four months into the study. When I connected with her there was something in the way. It felt like a big energy, like another person—the energetic presence of another person, and not a very nice person/energy. No matter what I tried, I could not get around this presence, nor could I reach my partner. So I decided to stay connected to whatever was going on and hold space for my partner. The presence never left. I finally stopped the session. I was curious as to what my partner's comments would be, as the presence did not feel good to me. She remarked that she had felt some strange and intense energy during the session. I explained what I had experienced and shared that I did not do anything, that I could not—that presence was in the way. I had never experienced this before, nor had my partner. We were left with a mystery; sometimes this happens. Since we are both TTers, we agreed to let each other know if we had another experience like this.

I notice for myself that distance TT is more intimate for me than physical TT. I feel a much more complete connection with the person. It is also a more intense experience of the altered state. It's as if the connection is more real than on the physical plane. If I am tired it can be a bit much for me, so I am cautious about when I engage in distance TT.

Practice with a Colleague

The practice suggested by this therapist can be an excellent strategy to prevent some of the pitfalls related above.

I think that the best thing I ever did was to spend a year with a Recognized Teacher colleague sharing Therapeutic Touch at a distance. Each week we met on Wednesday evening, ready for bed. We alternated weeks giving distance TT. We each wrote up our thoughts after the session (often the next day if we were receiving the session, since the healee always went to sleep afterward), and then on the weekend we shared our findings. Exchanging roles with a TT colleague in this way provides an incomparable opportunity to build sensitivity and confidence, as debriefing can be done at a depth not possible with an actual ill recipient.

This study allowed us both to learn to work at a distance with confidence and safety. I now (just in the last year) always start my distance Therapeutic Touch sessions with meditation before moving into the healing. By beginning with meditation I become grounded and centered.

When I teach distance healing I always suggest that my students buddy-up with someone to practice and share feedback, before trying it out on someone who is really ill. I also suggest "When in doubt, stop," and stress that our work is gentle, gentle, gentle.

I think the most important considerations for safe healing at-a-distance are lack of ego and confidence, which can be gained through practice with another healer who can give good feedback.

11

Healing-at-a-Distance
Resources for Further Study

Healing at-a-distance presents its own unique challenges. In addition to being difficult to verbally explain and quantify, the healer is sensorily deprived of feedback and connection with the healing partner. The entire process takes place in other realms. This study has barely scratched the surface. There are undoubtedly ways of exploring healing at-a-distance that we have yet to discover.

- Replications of present exploratory study.
- Multivariate research on practices of various cultures and their rituals for healing at-a-distance.
- Phenomenology of healing-at-a-distance practices and ceremonies of disparate religious groups.
- Longitudinal research on therapeutic effects of healing-at-a-distance practices.
- Quantitative studies of selected demographic variables among recipients of healing at-a-distance.
- Research on differential effects of healing at-a-distance when supplemented with musical variables, such as toning, harmonics, or polyphonic chanting.
- Multivariate research on synchronous happenings during healing-at-a-distance sessions.

- Research on the effects of healing at-a-distance and synchronous imagery by the healing partner.
- Qualitative study of the lived experience of the healer during healing-at-a-distance sessions.
- Development of criteria to assign level of faith or trust measures between healing partner and healer.

Editor's Note: Healing at-a-Distance in 2020

Healing at-a-distance increased dramatically in 2020 when the Covid-19 pandemic resulted in many people isolating and working from home. Zoom calls and other types of video chat connections with family, isolated elders, clients, and friends led some TT practitioners to experience surprisingly effective healing interactions online. Geographic distance, visual connection, or time zone differences do not seem to interfere with the effectiveness of the healing.

"Dennis," an experienced TT practitioner, participated in a hybrid teaching session where some were attending via Zoom and others were physically present, masked, and socially distanced. Just as for in-person groups, members held the intention for wholeness of the recipient. "I have never before done TT with people in Zoom land, while doing in-person TT," he said. "I am surprised, but I can feel all your energies. I had no idea it would be so powerful. Or that I would feel it so strongly."

TT teacher Lin Bauer commented: "Teaching via a virtual format such as Zoom is turning out to have some great advantages. People can attend from wherever they live in the world, guest presenters can pop in to teach certain sections, while attendees remain in the comfort of their own homes. And the group connections that develop during these classes are proving to be as deep as when we meet in person. Many practitioners have noted that they feel a heightened sensitivity while giving TT through Zoom, without the 'distraction' of the physical body, while feeling a deeper connection to their Inner Self. Both TT therapists and recipients have been amazed by the accuracy of the perceived cues, as well as the effectiveness of the

TT sessions. Dee had been telling us that we needed to find new ways to teach and reach out to people. I'm not sure she envisioned these exact circumstances, but she was very clear that technology would be a big part of the equation. And we got pushed into it faster than we would have without Covid-19, for sure."

A Suggested Bibliography for the Twenty-First Century

One of the most striking realizations of the "Healing-at-a-Distance Exploratory Study" is that the internal processing of healing at-a-distance most resembles intercessory prayer of traditional religions. Later, in reviewing our previous study, "'Looking Over My Shoulder,' A Study in Mindfulness," it was recognized that a distinct logical relationship could be seen between these two methods of healing. In considering the latter, one intuits that underlying this linkage there is a whole series of potential future-consciousness studies that will enhance insight into the subtle nature of the healing process itself. The present bibliography sets its sights on some current studies.

Two publications are particularly recommended—an exhaustive study on spiritual healing: Daniel J. Benor, M.D., *Spiritual Healing: Scientific Validation of a Healing Revolution* (Southfield, Mich.: Vision Publications, 2001); and J. A. Astin's systematic review of research up to the year 2000, cited below.

Abbot, N. C. "Healing as a Therapy for Human Illness: A Systemic Review." *Journal of Alternative and Complementary Medicine* 6, no. 2 (2000): 159–69.

Astin, J. A., E. Harkness, E. Ernst. "The Efficacy of Distant Healing: A Systemic View of Randomized Controlled Trials." *Annals of Internal Medicine* 132 (2000): 903–10.

Aviles, J. M., S. E. Whelan, D. A. Hernke, et al. "A Study of Intercessory Prayer and Cardiovascular Disease Progression in a Coronary Care Unit Population." *Mayo Clinic Proceedings* 76 (2001): 1192–98.

Baldaicchiao, D., and P. Draper. "Spiritual Coping Strategies: A Review of the Nursing Research Literature." *Journal of Advanced Nursing Practice* 34, no. 6 (2001): 833–41.

Brown, C. K. "Methodological Problems of Clinical Research into Spiritual Healing: The Healer's Perspective." *Journal of Alternative and Complementary Medicine* 6, no. 2 (2000): 171–76.

Browner, W. S., and L. Goldman. "Distant Healing: An Unlikely Hypothesis." *American Journal of Medicine* 108, no. 6 (2000): 507–8.

Charman, R. A. "Placing Healers, Healees, and Healing into a Wider Research Context." *Journal of Alternative and Complementary Medicine* 6, no. 2 (2000): 177–80.

Chibnall J. T., J. M. Jeral, and M. A. Cerullo. "Experiments on Distant Intercessory Prayer: God, Science, and the Lesson of Massah." *Archives of Internal Medicine* 161, no. 21 (2001): 1–13.

DeGracia, Donald J. Report of Referee on "The Effect of 'Healing with Intent' on Pepsin Enzyme Activity." *Journal of Scientific Exploration* 13, no. 2 (1999): 149–53.

Dossey, Larry. *Healing Words: The Power of Prayer and the Practice of Medicine.* Harper San Francisco, 1999.

———. "Prayer and Medical Science: A Commentary on the Prayer Study by Harris et al and a Response to Critics." *Archives of Internal Medicine* 160 (2000): 1735–38.

Harkness, E. F., N. C. Abbot, and E. Ernst. "A Randomized Clinical Trial of Distant Healing for Skin Warts." *American Journal of Medicine* 108 (2000): 448–52.

Hoover, D. R., and J. B. Margolick. "Questions on the Design and Findings of a Randomized Controlled Trial of the Effects of Remote Intercessory Prayer on Outcomes in Patients Admitted to the Coronary Care Unit." *Archives of Internal Medicine* 160, no. 2 (2000): 1875–76, discussion 1877–78.

Kaptchuk, T. "Distant Healing." *Archives of Internal Medicine* 134 (2001): 532–33.

Kiang, J., D. Marotta, M. Wurkus, and W. Jonas. "External Bioenergy Increases Intracellular Response to Heat Stress." *Journal of Investigative Medicine* 50, no. 1 (2002): 38–45.

Krieger, Dolores. *Therapeutic Touch as Transpersonal Healing.* Seattle, Wash.: SeaChange Health and Wellness, 2017.

Malmquist, J. "Scrutiny of Alternative Medicine—a Special Kind of Telemedicine." *Lakartidningen* 97 (2000): 51–52.

Matthews W. J., J. M. Conti, and S. G. Sireci, "The Effects of Intercessory Prayer, Positive Visualization, and Expectancy on the Well-Being of Kidney Dialysis Patients." *Alternative Therapies* 75, no. 5 (2001): 42–52.

Risch, K. I., E. Ernst, and J. Garrow. "A Randomized Controlled Study of Reviewer Bias against an Unconventional Therapy." *Journal of the Royal Society of Medicine* 93 (2000): 164–67.

Roberts L., I. Ahmed, and S. Hall. "Intercessory Prayer for the Alleviation of Ill Health." *Cochrane Database for Systemic Reviews* 2, no. 2 (1999).

Wiesendanger, H., L. Werthmuller, K. Reuter, and H. Walach. "Clinically Ill Patients Treated by Spiritual Healing Improve in Quality of Life; Results of a Randomized Waiting List–Controlled Study." *Journal of Alternative and Complementary Medicine* 7, no. 1 (2001): 45–51.

The Plausible Hunch
On the Possible Magic of Healing

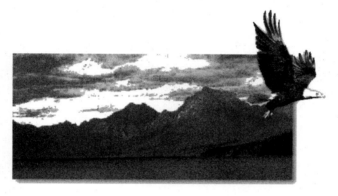

Healing is a window into a natural magic.
There it is,
a lump of wounded flesh,
and then touch,
Therapeutic Touch . . .

ABRACADABRAH!

Unseen clouds
Of inert biochemical molecules
Are drawn
In an uncanny manner
To the site of the wound,
Quietly
Sorting themselves out en route

To match
The needs of the damaged tissues.

As they approach
They move
On to

and then along
the fine, organic space lattices
of the injured tissues,
re-patterning
its constituents
as the healing mass proceeds
under the directive
of some prestigious Authority
whose dictates
no one questions.

Bit by bit
the molecules line up
according
to this apparently preconceived plan
Step by step
Balance and re-union occur,
Until—
EUREKA!
the healing is complete,
magically,
the tissue looks
As if never rent.
It is
of one piece;
wholing, haelen (healing)
has occurred!
Magic in the offing.

DOLORES KRIEGER

Acknowledgments

Nowhere would one know better that "it takes a village" than in the experience of bringing a manuscript into publication. Especially this one. Shortly before her death, our teacher and mentor, Dolores Krieger, appointed me editor of her final manuscript. She knew that I had a village behind me—and most especially, most particularly, that I would be supported by Dr. Pat Cole and Sandy Matheny, who had been at her side for more than a decade, developing and administrating the annual gatherings of the TT Dialogues, and also as dear friends.

Pat, Sandy, and I came together to form a "three-legged stool," as we referred to ourselves over the months of reading, rereading, conferring, writing, rewriting, and so on. I understand that a three-legged stool is the most stable structure on uneven ground, making it a good description of us and our process. For the three of us—as we joined with the international village of Therapeutic Touch in grieving our loss—this process of editing was facilitating our own healing, allowing us to maintain and celebrate our connection with Dee through her thoughts and words. Truly, these months of healing took us across uneven ground. But together, we forged a steady path. This final product would not have happened without Pat and Sandy.

For many years it was the tradition in Therapeutic Touch that Dora and Dee taught at Invitational Healers programs at Camp Indralaya, Orcas Island, Washington every June, and every July they did the same at Pumpkin Hollow Farm, Craryville, New York. After Dora's death in

1999, Dee continued this practice. In 2009 she decided that her traveling days were over. We should have noticed that she declared she was not in retirement, but rather "re-treadment," because in 2010 her next idea was to send out an invitation to members of the tribe with at least three-years' TT experience to come to Montana for a Dialogue on the Healing Moment. She told Sandy and Pat that she expected between six and eight people; it was a group of thirty who met that first year. Since then, over the decade there have been more than a hundred total attendees.

The Dialogues have produced the two studies included in this book, as well as the publication of *A Practice-Based Theory of Healing through Therapeutic Touch,* authored by Mary Anne Hanley, Ph.D., R.N., QTTT; Denise Coppa, Ph.D., FAAN, QTTT; and Deborah Shields, Ph.D., AHN-BC, QTTT. In their note these authors credit both Dee and "the expert TT practitioners who participated in the Montana Dialogues from 2010 to 2016, without whose insights and explorations this project would not have succeeded."

With the beginning of the incorporation process in 2011 as Therapeutic Touch Dialogues, Inc., came the formation of a board. Aside from Pat and Sandy, the board includes a number of dedicated Therapeutic Touch therapists and teachers:

Mary Anne Hanley, master synthesizer of huge swaths of information.
Lin Bauer, teacher and mentor par excellence.
Kathy Arquette, leader of Educational Kinesiology during breaks in working sessions at the Dialogues, with her considerable skill and engaging humor.
Linda Shockey and Marcia McEwen, videographers extraordinaire, who so capably undertook the task of recording the Dialogues each year.
Kathy Wilmering, overseer of archives. Additionally, Kathy is the publisher of Dee's *Therapeutic Touch as Transpersonal Healing,* for which Dee was very grateful.

Many thanks go out to all who participated in one or both of the studies, whose work is included in the book: Patricia Abrams, Kathy Arquette, Lin Bauer, Cheri Brady, Lynn W. Braillier, Sara Colburn, Pat

Cole, Allison Cooke, Pete Conlin, Sue Conlin, Bette Croce, Arlene Cugelman, Judy Custer, Stacey DeLuca, Jean Dunnett, Laura Dunning, Charlie Elkind, Jody Falconer, Cathy Fanslow, Sandra Flodin, Bev Forster, Peggy Frank, Rebecca Good, Chery Ann Hoffmeyer, Sharon Hunter, Debbie Lee, Sandy Matheny, Katherine Rosa, Lillian J. Ross, Nancy Sherk, Deb Shields, Mary Simpson, Dorothy Wood Smith, Betsy Ungvarsky, Kathy Wilmering, Paul Wolfe, and Bev Zabler.

We also acknowledge those qualified therapists, practitioners, and teachers throughout the international TT community who are currently serving as contacts for local and regional practice groups. These people may be contacted through TTIA and the Canadian networks (see Resources section, page 247).

United States
Florida: Kathy Barnett, Shirley Spear Begley
Illinois: Marilyn Johnston-Svoboda
Massachusetts: Catherine Collins
Montana: Pat Cole
New Hampshire: Elaine Wilk
New York: Sue Conlin, Susan Cutter
Ohio Heart of Healing
Oregon: Cordy Anderson, Lin Bauer, Linda Neal
Rhode Island: Anne M Porto, Sylvia Weber
Washington: Cindy Cole

Australia
New South Wales: Margaret Graham
Northern Territory: Susie Gregory
South Australia: Lainie Rawlins
Tasmania: Geoffrey Dunlop
Victoria: Jenny Cameron, Alina Gorris, Jane Hall, Virginnia Kingsford, Gerry Milton
Western Australia: Peta Nottle

Canada
Alberta: Chery Ann Hoffmeyer
Atlantic Provinces: Judy Donodvan Whitty
British Columbia: Tama Recker, Mary Lou Trinkwon
Manitoba: Tanya Sabourin
Ontario: Sheila Camp

France and Belgium
Eric Mazurier

Germany
Altdorf: Theresia Wilhelm
Berlin: Marita Petrak
Hamburg (and virtual): Heike Rahn
Kassel: Ria Rose
Rhein Main: Christina Müller-Stein
Virtual: Barbara Marcucci

Rwanda
Peninah Abatoni

Spain
Rosa Ferrer de Dios Larroya

Switzerland
Helen Chevalier

Turkey
Serbulent Bicer

United Kingdom
Karen Eastham, Annie Hallett

In addition, Therapeutic Touch has been taught in the following countries: Austria, Brazil, Czech Republic, Georgia, Iran, Japan, Kenya, Lesotho, Malawi, Netherlands, New Zealand, Norway, Russia, and Zimbabwe.

We are so grateful to all the people at Bear & Company who shepherded both the manuscript and our trio as we made our way through the publication adventure. It was on the frigid morning of February 4, 2019, that I was departing Kalispell, Montana, after a visit with Dee. While waiting on the plane during the de-icing of the wings, I saw on my phone that I had a reply from Jon Graham, acquisitions editor, to my query about this manuscript, saying that *yes,* Bear & Company was interested in publishing. As soon as I could, I let Dee know, and she was delighted. Jon's email was the initial communication that started us on our journey, and for a number of months he remained my touchstone.

Once we sent the manuscript to Bear & Company in May, we subsequently received emails from Patricia Rydle, assistant to the editor in chief, who gave us many important details about how to proceed. Later, catalog manager Erica Robinson contacted us with the cover design and catalog text.

We sensed the skillful presence of Jeanie Levitan, editor in chief, behind the scenes.

Manzanita Carpenter, publicist, provided us with important information about the marketing process.

Project editor Jamaica Burns reached out to us in the fall of 2020 with some entertaining thoughts and suggestions about the manuscript. The team experienced the kind of synchronicity that TT folk know well when freelance copy editor Abigail Lewis came on board. We were delighted to hear this from Abigail: "Dolores Krieger had a big impact on my life and has been helpful to me in my own healing, and also in working on my family." How wonderful to have a new pair of eyes overseeing the book, one with a background in TT. As Jamaica said, "I love it when the stars align and we get such a perfect team to shepherd a book through the editorial process!"

On every step of this journey I received help from both seen and unseen forces. Special thanks to Lin Bauer, who was always present at the other end of an e-mail to respond to questions and ruminations, no matter how goofy; to Sue Conlin, representing TTIA, who provided vital information in that capacity; and to my own longtime teaching partner, Peter Massey, R.N., who contributed eagle-eye proofreading.

Huge appreciation to David Spangler who so graciously contributed his foreword, which would have pleased Dee greatly. Thanks also to our gifted poet and artist-in-residence, Charlie Elkind, who contributed the images used in the book.

Part of Dee's legacy to the TT village lives on through her donation to the Therapeutic Touch Dialogues, Inc., of her home, the Rockery, and the surrounding forty acres of the Columbia Mountain Wildlife Sanctuary. We give thanks for the numerous caregivers who, with sensitivity and grace, attended Dee in her final weeks at her beloved Rockery. Appreciation also for support from her neighbors of many years, Ronnie and Doug Honthaas.

Last but not least, we extend gratitude beyond words to every member of our international TT village who is—so beautifully—on a daily basis, practicing, teaching, and living the vision of Dora Kunz and Dee Krieger into the twenty-first century. Deep bow to each one of you. *Namaste.*

Glossary

Note: Some of the terms herein are standard in classical spirituality or healing systems. Others are unique to TT and can be found in previous books by Dolores Krieger.

chakras: Translated from Sanskrit as "centers of consciousness whose structures are nonphysical," chakras are natural components of human-energy field dynamics that can transform universal energies into human energies. These subtle structures are reflected at the various levels of consciousness of the individual, but they have their source as universal fields of mind.

Deep Dee: A TT technique in which the therapist uses her own chakra complex to assess and come into resonance with the chakra complex of the patient, with the intention of assisting the vital-energy field of the patient to become more balanced.

deep listening: "Listening" through sentience when in sustained centering to hear not only one's words but the emotions underneath them. This may take the form of intuition or a vision or a sound that is "heard" but not through one's physical ears.

energy overload: Going beyond the point of balance of the healee's vital-energy field while in the process of directing healing energies. Reactions in the healee may include increased restlessness or signs of heightened irritability and intensified anxiety such as headache, nausea, hostility, anger, pain, or fear. Energy overload in the healee can be an indicator to the healer that she has not remained centered.

(the) Four Dragons: Exaggeration, fantasy, impulse, and wishful thinking. When the TT healer finds herself entering any of these states, she realizes she is not fully grounded and centered.

future consciousness: The state of becoming more percipient and informed about the possibilities of the future development of the TT process, and acting with discernment, compassion, spiritual drive, and purposeful engagement of the power of personal in-depth forces in this endeavor. Becoming more conscious about how the future quickens the human spirit, facilitates a creative shift in consciousness, and elevates the idea of self. In the process of enhancing such transformation in the individual, this shift in consciousness actualizes mental potential and moves us forward in our conceptualization of who we can be.

healing partner: It was implicit in TT from the beginning that the recipient was a partner in the healing process; indeed, any healing could not be effective without the permission—consciously and subconsciously—of the recipient. The healer and the healee are partners in the deepest sense. As time went by, "healing partner" became increasingly popular as an identifier for healee, client, patient, or recipient.

Inner Self: Refers to the timeless link between the personality and the spiritual; the Guide or Teacher. Characterized by quietude, peacefulness, clarity of mind, certainty, heightened confidence, joyfulness, and an abiding sense of inner strength.

intentionality: Not an emotion or personal desire but the much deeper force by means of which we focus ourselves—mind and body—to carry out a specific purpose.

inth: Sometimes used by TT therapists to describe the depth of their focus of attention. A human ultrasensorial dimension that transcends the three physical dimensions of length, width, and breadth. A fourth, energetic dimension where one "goes" during the experience of journeying inside oneself.

Issie: Some years ago, as part of a presentation at one of the mentorship programs at Camp Indralaya, Orcas Island, Washington, students began referring to the Inner Self—a term that had been adopted by

Dora Kunz—as IS, which evolved into the humorous and affectionate term "Issie." Dr. Krieger became fond of this nickname, and would often use it to playfully refer to Inner Self.

knowings: Not perceiving solely with the mind but from a multisensory state. Information may be sensed as a flash of intuition. The term is often applied to knowledge that comes suddenly, as a whole thought. Dee often referred to "knowing more than we can say."

prana: The Sanskrit term designating the potent energy flow that is used most often during the TT process and is the basis of all life fields. Prana is one of the most powerful energies in the vital-energy field; it vivifies, vitalizes, and animates all living beings. It can be conceived of as a nonphysical, energy-rich, unifying environment that interpenetrates every living cell and actuates its functions.

psychodynamic energy field: Traditionally referred to as the emotional field, this field interpenetrates each person's physical body and vital-energy flows. It is the bearer of such traits as sensory perceptions, reason, and the emotions. It is more permeable than the vital-energy field and can exhibit great elasticity, so that powerful discharges of feelings or thoughts dramatically enlarge the field.

scaffolding: The use by the TT therapist of her own centered and healthy subtle-energy fields as a model or template against which the healee can experience the repatterning of his own energy fields.

sentience: Sentience is the ability of an entity to have perceptual experiences or feelings. These experiences are subjective and transcend the physical/cognitive responses that humans have, such as creativity, intelligence, and intentionality. Sentience is an aspect of consciousness that cannot be measured, only described. It is a composite or product of sensory experiences and reflects the individual's ability to consciously experience these sensations. (With thanks to Denise Coppa.)

spiritual tension: The state in which the TT healer holds in her consciousness both the symptoms of disease or disorder and, simultaneously, her understanding of the potential for balance and wholeness. As the TT session progresses and the fields of the healee move toward balance, the tension is eased or released.

third eye: The sixth (ajna) chakra, with location designated between the eyebrows or slightly above, is the seat of the cognitive and subtle senses. The TT therapist may use this chakra during the assessment phase to visualize sites of imbalance in the healee's vital-energy field.

transpersonal: First coined by Carl Jung, as in "transpersonal/collective" unconscious. Describes the experience of a state of being beyond the usual range of the personality; it is characterized by a sense of being an integral part of a whole.

Transpersonal healing: This includes a variety of modalities that honor the whole person, seeking to assist in integration of all parts of the person. It also includes a perspective of each person being part of a greater whole.

TT blue: One of the colors that a TT therapist may use in the direction of energy toward the patient. The quality of the color is as if it is blue *light* able to interpenetrate the energy fields and the physical tissues of the healee. Visualizing this particular color has been found to be effective in situations of pain and anxiety. In keeping with the TT principle that there are no specific protocols and that each session is unique, TT therapists will make use of this color, other shades of blue, and combinations of colors to vary the intensity for a specific situation. Note Krieger's use of color on page 33.

unition: The action of joining together two or more things; the condition of being united.

universal healing field: There is a universal healing field in our cosmos; this seems to be the case since all living organisms have the capacity to heal themselves and, under the appropriate circumstances, to heal others also. The two main components of the field are order and compassion. The description of it varies with each person's individual experience and belief system. The universal healing field operates in Therapeutic Touch through the quiet moment of centering before we begin. We center ourselves by focusing within and thinking of peace. What we are really doing is feeling the peace and quiet of the Inner Self. Described by Dora Kunz in *The Spiritual Dimension of Therapeutic Touch*, 27–28.

unruffling: A way of modulating vital energies in the human energy field during the rebalance phase that addresses some of the disorder and imbalances in the vital-energy field. The therapist gently sweeps her hands through the field, intending the cues to change, dissolve, and move toward the periphery of the healee's field, where they can disperse.

vital-energy field: Vital energies are restless, shifting, rhythmic patterns in constant flow. These configurations of subtle energies are the basis for the physical functions, emotional and behavioral patterns, drive, thoughts, and intuitions that are uniquely encoded in each individual. The vital-energy field is the personal multidimensional space that surrounds and quickens each individual, energizing and reinvigorating her throughout life.

vivid visualization: Originally defined by Krieger, in *Living the Therapeutic Touch,* as "a spontaneous mental process in which a graphic pictorialization of an event arises to mind as if the visualizer is at the place of occurrence"—through the years this technique became more meaningful to her intuitive process in TT both for in-person and distance sessions. She found that the information in the field of the recipient that came to her through the vivid visualizations could impart deep meaning, and often insight, into the origins of the healee's condition. She would speak about suddenly receiving a "whole" picture or sense of an issue. This serves as an example of how one's intuitive knowing is continually evolving and growing on the path of Therapeutic Touch. Others may experience the deepening of their intuition in a myriad of ways. Krieger wrote extensively about vivid visualization in *Therapeutic Touch as Transpersonal Healing.*

Therapeutic Touch Resources

Therapeutic Touch Dialogues, Inc.

As Dolores Krieger wrote, "The aim of the Dialogues is to 'feel out' the future consciousness of Therapeutic Touch, both as a skilled healing practice and as an open-ended inner journey."

For more information about Therapeutic Touch Dialogues, Inc., contact

Pat Cole, M.D., QTTT
P.O. Box 393, Whitefish, MT 59937
info@ttdialogues.com

Therapeutic Touch International Association (TTIA)

Following the successful development by Dora Kunz and Dolores Krieger of the new healing modality, Therapeutic Touch (TT), in 1972, Dolores Krieger incorporated Nurse Healers Professional Associates, Inc., as a not-for-profit organization in New York State in 1979. A few years later, at the request of practitioners and teachers in other countries who were looking for guidance, we added the word "International" to our name. In 2005 we added a DBA designation of Therapeutic Touch International Association.

In 2020, as a response to the Covid-19 global pandemic, TTIA created many online programs for teaching and practicing TT and for gathering as a community of healers.

Please visit our website at
www.therapeutictouch.org
for more information about the practice and qualified TT practitioners and teachers, both online and in-person.

Therapeutic Touch Networks of Canada (TTNC)

The Therapeutic Touch Networks of Canada (TTNC), also known as Réseaux Toucher Thérapeutique du Canada (RTTC), was incorporated on January 17, 2011. A dynamic not-for-profit organization, dedicated to the promotion, practice, and acceptance of Therapeutic Touch as developed by Dora Kunz and Dolores Krieger, TTNC acts as the umbrella organization for all Canadian Therapeutic Touch networks, coordinating education, research, and communications with other international TT organizations.

For more information and to find recognized practitioners and teachers, visit
ttnc.ca

Index